'A valuable roadmap for our evolution a‹
of practical advice in a positive tone tha
unspoken in our profession.'

— *Lizzie L*

'This book is an invaluable resource for all yoga teachers and mentors. Jess offers us a framework for established and emerging protocols regarding the craft of teaching yoga. In clear and lucid language, she expresses some very complex teaching strategies, highlights common pitfalls encountered by yoga professionals, and offers numerous exercises to help teachers find clarity to enter the field with confidence.'

*— Greg Nardi, Owner of Ashtanga Yoga Worldwide and
Co-founder of Amayu Yoga*

'With insight and wisdom, Jess skilfully and sensitively invites us to reflect on our path, offering the tools of inquiry with which to do so. Everything an aspiring or experienced yoga teacher wishes they'd known, things they hadn't thought to consider plus plenty more to contemplate and ponder.'

*— Dina (Medina) Cohen, Yoga and Mindfulness Educator,
Mentor and Teacher Trainer*

'This friendly handbook provides an essential companion for new yoga teachers embarking on their first teaching steps. Written not only from her own experience but also that of her peers, Glenny gives the inside scoop on how to "keep on keeping on" in this new and daunting world of yoga teaching.'

— Rebecca French, YogaLondon

'An extremely useful book full of practical advice for yoga teachers at all stages of their teaching journey. It covers issues that are both perennial and up to date, from being clear about financial agreements to handling consent in adjustments. Timely, accessible and sensitive to diverse needs and situations.'

— Theo Wildcroft, PhD

'In a rapidly changing yoga world, this is a very valuable resource, full of common-sense pieces of practical advice otherwise often only learned through trial and – frequently – error. As important for those who have been teaching for years as it is for those just starting out.'

– Dr Graham Burns, Yoga Teacher and Teacher Trainer

'This wonderful book is rich with guidance and practical advice for new and trainee teachers, and is equally inspiring for experienced teachers. Jess has woven together many areas of expertise in a generous, warmly presented, very accessible way. It's like having Jess, with all her years of experience, in the room with you as you practice, plan or teach. Highly recommended.'

– Jane Sleven, 37 years extensive Hatha and Ashtanga Yoga Teaching Experience in UK and Internationally

'An invaluable guide, Jess's book is clearly written and informative. Packed with practical exercises and advice, it offers realistic and wise counsel in navigating the range of common, yet tricky, situations faced by yoga teachers every day.'

Catherine Annis, Senior Yoga Teacher and Founder of Intelligent Yoga Teacher Training

The Yoga Teacher Mentor

The YOGA
Teacher Mentor

A Reflective Guide to Holding
Spaces, Maintaining Boundaries,
and Creating Inclusive Classes

JESS GLENNY

Foreword by Norman Blair

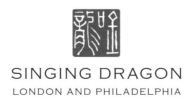

SINGING DRAGON
LONDON AND PHILADELPHIA

First published in 2020
by Singing Dragon
an imprint of Jessica Kingsley Publishers
73 Collier Street
London N1 9BE, UK
and
400 Market Street, Suite 400
Philadelphia, PA 19106, USA

www.singingdragon.com

Library of Congress Cataloging in Publication Data
A CIP catalog record for this book is available from the Library of Congress

British Library Cataloguing in Publication Data
A CIP catalogue record for this book is available from the British Library

ISBN 978 1 78775 126 2
eISBN 978 1 78775 127 9

Printed and bound in Great Britain

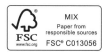

MIX
Paper from
responsible sources
FSC® C013056

आचार्यात् पादमादत्ते पादं शिष्यः स्वमेधया
पादं सब्रह्मचारिभ्यः पादं कालक्रमेण

A student receives a quarter [of their knowledge] from the teacher, a quarter from their own intelligence, a quarter from fellow students and a quarter in the course of time.

Sanskrit saying[1]

Contents

Foreword

I first met Jess Glenny – the author of this much-needed book – in 2002. Since then we have had many discussions and exchanged many tips for yoga teaching and yoga teacher mentoring.

Jess is a practitioner who speaks her mind. She is not frightened of ploughing her own furrow. She is a teacher of courage and intelligence. A person who stands up for what she believes in. A practitioner who knows this truth: 'Just regular humans being human.' A writer who draws on vast wells of her own experience. Her first yoga class was at the start of the 1980s. As she writes: 'In 1981…yoga was deeply untrendy.'

Rather than following the crowds, Jess uses tools of insight and empathy to explore paths of integrity and understanding. Instead of 'a culture obsessed with looking, staying and feeling young', here the questions at the heart of Jess's teachings – and this book – are more like: 'What imprisons us and what frees us?'

The Yoga Teacher Mentor is grounded in exploring what can make us better yoga teachers. Sometimes, certain things that are difficult or challenging have to be said – and Jess is a person (as this book clearly shows) who can say them. Weaving webs from her own personal experiences, stories from others and wider social/psychological/structural issues, this is a thoughtful and practical book.

Being supported is important. Whether this is called 'mentoring', 'supervision' or 'peer groups', we all need helping hands. Many other people-centred fields – like yoga teaching – have this support as a non-negotiable requirement. The truth is this can be the difference between sinking and swimming, the difference between collapsing in a heap and being grounded, the difference between unethical actions and maintaining integrity. Receiving advice and skilful guidance from more experienced teachers is a precious gift. This book is such a gift.

Teaching yoga has plenty of pitfalls and problems: the yoga studios that can be more like supermarkets; the teacher as a rock star; the students wanting to be 'fixed'; people-pleasing; grumpy moods; injured bodies; the inevitable ups and downs of class numbers; the certainty of challenges. These are common experiences amongst yoga teachers, as are the beauties, joys and significant responsibilities. In Jess's words: 'Teaching yoga is a job…a practice, a vocation and a journey of becoming.'

What makes a good yoga teacher? Reading – and re-reading – this book can be one of the paths towards becoming better and more skilled teachers. This book is not about Facebook likes. Nor is it about ticking boxes and getting Continuing Professional Development points. It is not about deluding ourselves. Rather, this book is about evolving and exploring yoga teaching. It pulls down the pretences and undermines the projections. These pages contain strong statements that we can all benefit from studying – whether we have been teaching yoga for two weeks or 20 years, whether we are training to be teachers or thinking about training.

I hope that this book informs and inspires you, guides your teaching and encourages you to take practical steps that help you become a better yoga teacher. Both newly qualified teachers and those who have taught thousands of classes will find material here that is relevant and thought-provoking.

The Yoga Teacher Mentor will challenge you, constructively confuse you, amuse you, and cause both despair and joy. The Yoga Teacher Mentor is readable, accessible and – in my opinion – essential.

Norman Blair, senior yin yoga teacher, yoga teacher mentor
and author of *Brightening Our Inner Skies: Yin and Yoga*

Acknowledgements

Thanks go first and foremost to all my yoga teacher mentees, apprentices and assistant teachers, who provided the context, impetus and much of the background material for this book.

Thanks also to members of Yoga Teachers UK, Yoga Teachers Support and Mentoring, and Yoga Teacher Elders Co-mentoring and Support for generously responding to my endless questions about your teaching experiences and generally broadening the scope of this book. You can find these groups on Facebook.

Thanks to all my wonderful students, who provide me with ongoing opportunities to hone my teaching skills, encounter new challenges and evolve my teaching 'container'. Learning and teaching really is a two-directional process.

I'm very grateful to my friend and colleague Norman Blair, who spurred me to turn the written material created for my yoga teacher mentor groups into this book. Without Norm's encouragement I probably wouldn't have believed there was a book in all of this.

Thanks also to Maitripushpa Bois, who has been generous in offering advice on contracts, permissions and other publishing practicalities.

Finally, thanks to the editorial team at Jessica Kingsley Publishers for creating a beautiful book with great production values – and also for making the publication process easy and pain-free for this autistic writer.

Namaste!

A Note on the Case Histories

The case histories in this book are all fictionalised amalgamations of different experiences of different teachers in mentoring. I hope and expect you will notice many similarities with experiences of your own; however, any resemblance to real teachers and real students is only that. No actual teachers or students are represented in the case histories and the first names used are all made up. Advice and suggestions offered by experienced teachers and studio owners are likewise mixed up, fictionalised and anonymised. Direct quotations of real people are given with the person's full (first and second) name.

Introduction

Welcome to *The Yoga Teacher Mentor*. This book is about the *practice* of teaching yoga. It's about how to hold people in the experience of yoga, and how to support yourself as you engage in this rich, complex, often challenging but always rewarding process – because there's a lot more to being a yoga teacher than alignment and sequencing.

This book grew out of material I originally created for the yoga teacher mentor groups I run in South East London. This material has been supplemented by input from my one-to-one mentees, and from yoga teachers in several social media support and mentoring groups. I'm very, very grateful to all of you for your contributions: for your stories and experiences, from the sad to the hilarious through the thought-provoking and mind-changing; for your perspectives, often different from my own; and for continually informing me about the range of issues yoga teachers come up against while working in a variety of settings and styles, some of them outside my own personal experience.

Once you start reading, you'll probably notice that many of the themes overlap and overflow individual chapters. How we hold space as yoga teachers, what constitutes healthy and mutually sustaining boundaries, the meaning of safety in a yoga class, how we create generative relationships with our students... These kinds of questions will arise again and again in a variety of contexts. I hope that seeing them through different lenses will help to amplify your understanding and expand your sense of what may be an appropriate response in different situations.

Experienced yoga teachers rarely talk in terms of right and wrong, and that's not what this book sets out to do either. The intention is to invite, offer possibilities, suggest and signpost. There are no prescriptions for the perfect yoga teacher, and there are few absolute prohibitions. We probably all know yoga teachers who appear to break every rule in the book and yet teach fabulous classes founded in true integrity. Shena Grigor of MadDogYoga says:

> I'm sure people have come to my class, not liked it and gone elsewhere. I swear a lot when I'm teaching. It's part of me. There's lots of cheeky banter, teasing and cheering from everyone, and it can often sound more like a pub. I frequently highlight different students who have found something beautiful in a posture or executed something well. They are not necessarily the most 'advanced' or the most flexible but those who have achieved something new for them, and yes, other students clap. People sometimes take the piss or gently push others over (me included); however, the class does have structure and is not a free-for-all. There's no feeling of jealousy or one-up-manship, just genuine fondness and caring for each other, and concern if someone is ill, has to go into hospital, loses a spouse, or something like that. People are chatty and socialise a lot out of class, even though they only met through yoga. There's great community spirit.

This kind of teaching grows out of the fabric of the person. It is truly authentic and cannot be imitated. On the face of it, it may appear to contravene generally accepted teaching boundaries, but in fact the teacher has a strong internal locus of ethics[1] that ensures the well-being of their students.

For a long time, these words, from senior ashtanga vinyasa teacher Richard Freeman, have been at the crux of the mentor programmes I facilitate for yoga teachers:

> It is the teacher's foremost duty to give you back your intelligence, to return you to your heart, to encourage you to access yourself. They do this by being who they really are and by being completely honest and compassionate with you.

This is a tall order, but teaching yoga is a challenging profession – a vocation, not a lifestyle choice. We cannot teach well without an ongoing commitment to self-practice, self-study and full engagement in the experience of being in relationship with our students. None of this is for the casual or faint-hearted.

I hope that you will be inspired, challenged, stimulated and supported by the material you find in this book, and that it will help you to be a more authentic, sensitive and capacious teacher. *Namaste!*

1

Where Have You Come From, Where Are You Now, and Where Do You Want to Go?

This chapter is about trajectories. It's about the disparities that can sometimes arise between the direction our head is taking and where our body wants to go. It's about our hopes and what may prevent us from living into them, and about our fears and how they may be limiting us. It's also about the process of becoming a teacher and the different phases of development we move through as we expand our capacity to hold people in practice.

Setting your compass

This first chapter is a little different from those that follow. It begins with a substantial piece of experiential work for exploring where you find yourself now on your teaching path. We will be working somatically – through the body – so that rather than reflecting on where you *think* you are, you can access your *embodied* awareness of your current position, and of any direction that may be emerging.

When I facilitate mentor groups, the first session always consists of this or a similar experiential process – and most sessions include a piece of somatic work. The majority of people come to mentoring with lots of questions. Most of the time I hold back on giving my own answers to these, and I discourage other mentees from offering opinions. What I do try to do is provide opportunities for mentees to access their own internal compass so that they can emerge their own path. Each person's pathway is unique to them – and might be a blind alley to another teacher. When we proceed in this way from an embodied source of feeling, knowing and orienting, we discover a natural depth and authority in our teaching that is a unique expression of who we are.

REFLECTION

Offer some attention to where you are now in your yoga journey. Include both your personal yoga practice and your teaching. Let this be a meditation. Allow the point of your attention – the place you are witnessing yourself from – to drop back from your forehead, and allow your attention to float. Rather than thinking about what you know, open your awareness to feelings, words, images and sensations that may be different from those your cognitive mind anticipates. Whatever comes, allow it in.

- How did you get to here? Were there moments of inspiration, key events, teachers, trainings, meetings, initiations?

- If you could move in any direction, where would you go? Loosen yourself from any practical considerations. What would it look like if there were no limitations? What are your cherished hopes and dreams?

- Where do you feel you are actually being taken? Is this congruent with where you deeply desire to go?

EXPERIENTIAL WORK: MY HOUSE

You can make this exploration alone or together with a yoga teacher friend or friends. Don't read in advance beyond step 4 of 'Drawing the house' - you will spoil the big reveal and skew the exploration!

You will need:

- About 90 minutes in a quiet space with a little room to move around in - somewhere you will not be interrupted. Allow an extra half-hour or so if you're working with others.

- A yoga mat, blanket or soft surface, plus any props you like to use.

- A poster-sized piece of paper (I usually use flipchart paper).

- Crayons, pencils, pastels or any other drawing materials you find inviting.

- A notepad and pen.

- Optional: a clock, watch or timer.

Entering the terrain of your body

We start this exploration with a little gentle, supine yoga. You could equally well dance in an improvised way, or do another practice in which your body leads and your thinking mind takes a back seat. I tend to start with yoga because it's familiar to yoga teachers and so feels safe at a first meeting, when we don't yet know each other very well, but you can do something different if you prefer. The exploration will work best if you avoid anything technical or alignment-based, in which your body has to follow a pre-set structure. This is about your body choosing and the rest of you following.

Any time you are invited to centre in your body during the course of this book, you can use this short process.

1. Choose three passive, lying-down postures that you really enjoy and can stay in with ease for about five minutes. Three that I often do are chest opening over a bolster, supine twist and child's pose over a bolster, but you can do different ones if you prefer. Include any props you need to make yourself feel as comfortable as possible.

2. Lie down on your mat. Let your body settle into the floor... Allow the floor to take all of your weight. Let any expression dissolve out of your face...allowing your mouth to soften...including your tongue and the roof of your mouth... Let the hinges of your jaw relax... Imagine that the tough fibrous joints of your skull slightly soften so that your skull can be a little less pressed together than it might otherwise be.

3. Bring your attention to your breath. There's no need to change it in any way; just notice it. If it changes on its own, follow. You might notice where you feel your breath moving (nostrils, rib cage, diaphragm, belly...); what the quality of your breath is like (deep, shallow, slow, fast, fluid, ragged...); whether your breath is flowing freely everywhere or whether there are places that it doesn't go, and so on.

4. Allow your attention to expand so that as well as breath you include sensations. What is your physical experience in this moment?

Track any shifts and changes. You can move towards any physical sensation or away from it. The intention is to keep finding the sweet spot where you can stay calmly aware of what's happening. If you start to feel spaced out, panicky or overwhelmed, take a mental step back. If that doesn't enable you to re-find equilibrium, come back to your breath, or to an awareness of your body in contact with the floor, or to the sounds around you now, or open your eyes and orientate yourself to the room you are in now.

5. Allow your attention to expand so that as well as breath and sensations you include any emotions you are aware of. How are you feeling? What does the emotional landscape look like? Include both what is so familiar it's like furniture, and what is new and surprising. Pay particular attention to anything that seems to you ridiculous, inappropriate or not allowed. These responses may mark entry points to potential new awareness. Remember to stay where you can be fully present. You can choose to move away from any experience that is overwhelming or makes you want to zone out.

6. Allow your attention to expand so that as well as breath, sensations and emotions you include any thoughts you are aware of. How is your mind in this moment? Busy, quiet, compressed, full, empty, fuzzy...? You might notice what kinds of messages your mind is sending you at the moment, including any tone of voice. If you become entangled in the skeins of a story, notice...and simply return to witnessing.

7. Breath, sensations, emotions and thoughts are constantly changing. Let your attention shift to the part of you that does not change in this way. In the traditional Buddhist analogy, breath, sensations, emotions and thoughts are compared to clouds. Sometimes they are few, sometimes they are many, but behind them, whether we can see it or not, the sky is always present, always clear. You may think of this 'sky' part of you as soul, Buddha nature, *atman* or essential self, or you may understand it as the genetic knot that tethers all your you-things to you. Notice what's there when you witness from the perspective of this place.

8. Enter your first posture. You are going to rest here for about five minutes. Without fixing your attention, allow it to include some awareness of where you are now in your yoga-teaching life and the direction you would like to take. Let your attention come and go.

Include breath, sensations, emotions and thoughts, whether they seem to be relevant to your teaching or not. When the five minutes is up, rest in *savasana* for a few breaths.

9. If your posture has two sides, now enter the second side, or move on to your second posture. Hold for about five minutes. Continue to rest your awareness in all of your experience, with a particular curiosity about where you are now and where you would like to go as a teacher. When five minutes is up, rest in *savasana* for a few breaths.

10. Continue like this until you have moved through both sides of all three of your postures. End with a brief *savasana*.

Drawing the house

Make sure you allow plenty of quiet, empty transition space between the steps in this exploration. Move slowly and give yourself time to integrate each stage.

1. Allow 10 minutes for this step. Gather your paper and crayons. Make sure you continue drawing until 10 minutes is up (even if you think you've finished), and make sure you stop as soon as the time is up. Use a clock, watch or timer if you like. You are going to draw the basement of a house. This is your house, but it isn't any house you actually live in (although aspects of your real home may be present). You can include the area around the basement (garden, path, pavement/sidewalk, fence). You can include windows and doors. You can draw the contents of the basement. Your drawing can be realistic or impressionistic or abstract. Use whatever colours you are drawn to. There are no rules about how this should look or what to include or leave out. Draw from your felt experience. Don't pause. Even if you don't know what's coming next, keep a crayon moving on your sheet of paper. These moments of not knowing are often the most potent: they make space for body-mind to come through.

2. Allow 10 minutes for this next step. Draw the main part of the house. It may have a kitchen, bedrooms, living rooms, bathrooms, a yoga room. It may be like nothing that could exist in reality or it could include elements of a building or buildings you actually know. Feel what needs to be there. Don't stop to think – draw!

3. Allow 10 minutes for this next step. Draw the roof and attic spaces. You can also include the sky and anything on the roof. There may be clouds, birds, chimneys, the sun. Let your imagination run riot. Anything is allowed.

4. Take some time to look at your completed picture. What is your general impression? Do you like it? Does it disturb you? Is it colourful or monochrome? Is it mostly curves or mostly lines or a mixture of both? Is it realistic? Pure fantasy? What do you notice?

5. Now be aware that:

   i. The basement is where you have come from as a yoga teacher. This is your soil, your roots.

   ii. The main living area - the body of your house - is where you are now.

   iii. The roof space is what you are moving towards - your plans, your aspirations, and perhaps where you are headed if you don't make changes.

   Knowing this, what do you see now? Are some areas more filled in than others? What colours and shapes have you used and where? Were some sections easy to envisage and others less so? Do you have a secure foundation? What is your relationship with it? What's happening in your daily living space now? Is this how you would like it to be? What does your trajectory (your roof space) look like? You may want to make a note of anything that strikes you or feels significant.

6. If you could change your present (living area) and your direction (roof space) in any way, how would that be? Go ahead and do it. Notice how it feels to make the changes and how they affect your whole picture. Again, if you find it helpful, make notes of anything that feels important.

7. If you are doing this exploration with a friend or friends, now split into pairs. One of you is the speaker, the other is the listener. (You will be changing over later.) If you're an odd number, the third person is the witness.

   i. The speaker has five minutes to talk about any aspect of their experience of this exploration they would like to share in words.

It's fine to choose not to share some things, but don't hold back unnecessarily. If you want to, you can show your picture.

ii. The listener simply listens. No verbal responses are allowed.

iii. The witness (if there is one) witnesses the whole interaction without saying anything. They are the space-holder.

If the speaker runs out of things to say before their five minutes is up, then you sit together in silence. (This is great practice for the foundational yoga teacher skill of sitting quietly with a student.) If you still have more to say when your five minutes is up, save it for later. This is not a conversation. Don't interrupt the speaker, prompt them, comment on what they say or fill any silent spaces with talk. (This is great practice for the foundational yoga teacher skill of listening to your student without interrupting or expressing an opinion.) If you are the speaker, do not ask the listener or witness what they think or elicit comments from them.

When five minutes is up, thank each other by bringing your hands to prayer position and bowing. Then swap roles. Repeat and swap for a third time if you're a three.

Anything that is shared is confidential. If you want to talk later to one of your partners about something you have said, that's fine, but don't ask one of your partners about something they said. What each person spoke about belongs to them.

Moving forward

Keep your picture and look at it from time to time. As your perspective shifts and changes, so will what you see. Your picture is a dynamic resouce for reflecting on:

- The grounding you already have - where it's strong and where it needs to be fortified.

- Your aspirations - where you are limiting yourself versus where you may need a reality check.

- Your true trajectory - where you are headed and whether this is congruent with where you deeply desire to go.

- Any other information your picture yields to you.

You can use your picture as a basis for more practical discussions about ways forward, but don't forget to keep referring back to your felt sense of direction - what your body knows. Let yourself be informed by this stranger, deeper and more mysterious compass.

Phases of becoming[1]

Teaching yoga is a job requiring additional skills in administration, marketing, budgeting and PR, but it's also a practice, a vocation and a journey of becoming. Like Bunyan's Christian,[2] on this pilgrim's progress we encounter a set of metaphysical landmarks: the Slough of Despond ('I'll never be a decent yoga teacher'), the Valley of Humiliation ('How could I have forgotten half of that sun salutation?!'), the Hill of Lucre ('I really want 30 students in my class… I really want 30 students in my class…!'), and the Celestial City ('I'm so, so lucky to be making a living from something I passionately love!'). Traversing these terrains brings us depth, knowledge and capacity as a teacher. It enables us to relate to our students not just as someone who knows about yoga, but as a human being with the ability to safely navigate the full range of our human experiences.

In the process of becoming a yoga teacher, we move through a series of stages pretty much universal to everyone who has ever undertaken the teaching journey. As a beginning teacher, you may feel as if you are the only person who ever felt paralysed or physically sick with nerves before a class, but this is a common experience, as is, ultimately, the sense of coming home to teaching as a place of comfort and repose.

1. Survival mode

I'm a teacher in training. Yesterday I did the first class in my teaching practice. I was really, really nervous. I forgot all sorts of things. There were some complete beginners, and I know I should have given them modifications for some postures, but there just wasn't time. There were six people, and it felt so difficult to keep track of all of them and take care of their needs. I don't feel at all confident and am thinking about giving up on my dream of becoming a yoga teacher. I just don't think I can do this.

Carol

When we first start to teach, our main objective is to get out of each class alive. We are completely overwhelmed by the amount of things we have to manage all at the same time. We can't remember the names of the postures (or of the students). We don't know which way to face, how to cue movement in words, or how to adjust students back into functional movement when we see postures going haywire. Time seems to slow down ('How will I ever fill 30 minutes?') and then speed up ('Shit! I haven't got time for *savasana*!'). This is completely normal.

It all looks so easy when a seasoned teacher does it, and there's a reason for this. When an experience is already known, the human brain is able to remember it without having to think. This is known as 'implicit memory'. There's an effortless quality to implicit memory. For example, it's easy to remember that Friday comes after Thursday (implicit memory), because we experience the progression of days every week. If you've counted a sun salutation in Sanskrit twice a week for two years, this, too, will have become an implicit memory, and the numbers will surface in sequence, with the relevant breath, without any need for conscious thought. Many of our implicit memories are 'procedural', that is to say, they are motor memories, such as riding a bike, making a cup of tea, following a route from home to the local station, or adjusting *parivrtta parsvakonasana*.

In a led ashtanga class, I might be counting the posture in Sanskrit for the whole class, giving verbal feedback to an individual student, adjusting them physically, noticing that a couple of people are struggling and need help from the assistant teacher, and glancing at the clock to check that we're on track… simultaneously and without feeling flustered. Much of what an experienced teacher does in a yoga class, they have done hundreds and hundreds of times. They are no longer wasting thought on it, and this frees them up to do many things competently at the same time. If, as a beginning teacher, you keep on keeping on, you, too, will begin to encode experiences in implicit memory. Everything in your class will start to slow down and become more spacious and you will have time to notice what's happening and to consider your responses.

The more aspects of teaching you have already stored in implicit memory when you come to teach your first class, the easier it's going to be. If you already teach in a different capacity, for example, you won't need to think so much about some of the skills related to holding the class container: making the group feel comfortable, gearing your material to the ability of the group, holding authority while still being friendly and accessible, and so on.

One way to ensure that you already have a body of experience when you start to teach your own class is to apprentice with or assist a senior teacher. If you're experimenting with a verbal cue or practising an adjustment (one you have been taught and are competent to try) as an apprentice in someone else's class, you can concentrate purely on the cue or on the adjustment without having to keep all the other plates spinning. It's very tough to step into your first class as a teacher without any transferrable experience, so if you can apprentice or assist, do. Aside from the teaching practice, the mentoring and feedback you will receive will be invaluable. You will also be building strong relationships within the local teaching community you are about to enter. (For more on apprenticing and assisting, see Chapters 2 and 9.)

2. Comfort and competency

The development of some measure of comfort and competency when teaching a class is usually accompanied by a huge sense of relief. At this stage, we still need to rely quite heavily on the structures, forms and parameters we have been given by our own teachers, but as long as we stick with these, we are able to teach a sound, basic class to a group of people with no particular health conditions or injuries. We are not yet able to improvise all that much, and if something out-of-the-box happens, we may be thrown. For this reason, a teacher at this stage will still need quite a bit of mentoring and supervision.

The most useful form of professional development in this phase is usually teaching, teaching and more teaching. This is a time for applying and integrating the basic skills you have learnt rather than adding more complex ones. A key skill is knowing your limitations. In this phase, students with health issues other than very run-of-the-mill ones are best referred to an experienced or specialist teacher.

3. Creativity

The transition to this phase is usually made after a few years of regular teaching. This is where we start to make the material we are teaching our own. We emerge our own particular style and orientation to what we are teaching. We may diverge from the structures we were taught and create original forms, drawing from many diverse sources of inspiration. We can flow with whatever happens in the class and weave it into our teaching, and may start to bring more humour and idiosyncrasy into our approach.

Making the transition to creative teaching requires some audacity. As yoga teacher Lizzie Lasater says:

> To teach out of your own experience takes courage. It's a form of honesty to offer your students an idea or movement or sequence that you didn't receive from your teachers but instead developed in the laboratory of your own practice. But that's where it gets interesting. That's where it becomes juicy and wild and unknown. That's exactly where I want to live.[3]

This is a time when we may look for specialist or more advanced training, and we may notice particular directions emerging (for example, working with cancer, mindfulness approaches, creating choreographic flows, and so on).

4. Home

I was doing a facilitator training in a new discipline – an allied form of movement. A few of us were already very experienced teachers, but most were completely new to teaching. Came the day, near the end of the first residential module, when we were all asked to teach a short session for a small group of fellow trainees. Around me, all were freaking out! When it was my turn to take the teacher role, a profound sense of calm came over me. It was like a deep exhalation. After all the topsy turvy of being in a different city, with different people, a different bed, a different routine and a shed-load of information to assimilate, this was a known place, one of confidence and comfort, where I could step into myself, relax and be home. It was like putting on my favourite pair of slippers.

Allie

When teaching starts to feel like home to us – when we go there to feel centred, grounded, familiar and at ease – we have become a seasoned and flavoursome teacher. This threshold is often reached somewhere around the 10-year mark.

In this phase, we are often working with the bigger picture. Yoga becomes the way in which we relate to other people and to our environment rather than a series of postures. While a newer teacher may also understand this intellectually, they are in the professional phase of building structure, establishing basic skills, and creating style and identity, and are in most cases not yet capable of teaching from this expanded perspective, as the elder yoga teacher does in an effortless and organic way.

At this stage we are also usually a mentor (formally or informally) for newer teachers. We may run trainings, write books or articles, and hold positions of responsibility in professional organisations. We are respected in our professional communities, and our views are sought out and taken seriously.

Being where you are

It's simply not possible to skip the foundation phases and land immediately in being at home as a teacher. As an essential part of our process of growth and development, we are called on to tolerate feelings of out-of-control, inadequacy and not knowing what to do or whether we are getting it right. Experiencing any of these feelings is not a problem; it's a sign that we are engaged in learning and in accumulating valuable experience. And even the at-home teacher sometimes feels unsure, incompetent and out of their depth. For this teacher, though, such feelings are old and familar friends. They are able to welcome them, invite them in, sit down with them while they spill their tea and eat all the biscuits, then wish them well as they rise and depart again. No drama, just regular humans being human.

REFLECTION

- Which phase of the teaching journey are you in? What are the challenges associated with this phase? What are the good bits?

- Have you experienced any 'dark nights of the soul' – times when you felt like giving up on teaching yoga? How did you come through these? If you are in one now, what does it feel like? What are your doubts and fears? You might like to draw these or free-write about them (writing whatever comes into your head, without stopping, whether it makes sense or not).

- Imagine yourself in five years' time. Who do you imagine you will be as a teacher then? What will you be teaching and to whom? What sort of roles will you have within your student and teaching communities?

2

Setting Out

In this chapter we will be looking at some of the practical issues, learning edges and ethical dilemmas involved in entering the field as a yoga teacher. How do you make the transition from student/trainee/practitioner to professional yoga teacher? What are some of the pitfalls? What are the key things you need to know?

The teacher-explorer

I've just qualified and am setting up my first classes as a yoga teacher – but I'm so aware of my limitations. I know I need to publicise my classes, but I also want to make my beginner's mistakes quietly and unostentatiously. I live in a small community where everyone knows each other and it's hard to be anonymous. How do I keep my teaching and learning separate?

Dot

It can be daunting to set out your stall as a yoga teacher. For most people, becoming a teacher involves stepping into a new, and perhaps long-dreamed-of, identity. This can be exciting, but it also often brings up feelings of fear and inadequacy. It can feel as if you are putting yourself very publicly on the line, and you may wonder whether you are really 'good' enough.

One way to view a teacher is as a person with superior knowledge whose role is to impart that knowledge to the student, a person with little or no knowledge, an empty vessel who passively receives the teaching. In this paradigm, the teacher is presumed to have authority over the material they are teaching and may also be endowed with authority over the students. Some of us may have imprinted this model for the teacher–student relationship from our own schooling. However, it poorly serves teachers of present-day practitioners, people with diverse life experiences and many transferable skills, whose primary need is holding through somatic process (the investigation of their own embodied experience). As senior ashtanga vinyasa teacher David Garrigues says:

> Knowledge is not something to be dictated and enforced from outside. The student is already in possession of their own way to walk towards truth, and therefore the teacher is careful to provide structure without rigidity, and flexibility in adhering to collective rules. The teacher values the innate drive and intelligence of the student and wants to know what lights the student's fire – and responds spontaneously and creatively to help the student become stronger in forging her own independent path.[1]

Teaching yoga requires us to be pliable, vulnerable and willing to enter into the realm of not-knowing with our students. A small part of teaching is instruction: conveying cognitive information. By far the greater part is open-ended exploration. In this process, it's not possible to keep our teaching and our learning separate – because they are not two different things. Teaching is a practice, and a teacher is always also a student of their art, always pressing out into places where they are no longer sure of the reason, the route or the meaning. Neither is it possible to be anonymous here. As a yoga teacher, we are called upon to stand behind and own our learning within the community of our peers and students. In this engagement lies the ground of our authenticity. A teacher has to be willing to be seen, felt and heard – because if we are not, our students cannot find us, and they will not feel held by our presence.

Don't expect to know everything as a teacher (or think that anyone else expects you to). Curiosity and an open mind, not omniscience, are the qualifications for the job. 'I don't know' is a great response to a student's question. It helps to frame the teacher–student relationship as one in which you are accompanying your student in a process of investigation – rather than imparting pre-formed truths to them as an expert – and reinforces for them that their learning process is unique and their own. As teacher, writer and education activist Parker Palmer says, 'A good teacher does not so much fill the space as open it up for others.'[2] (For more on giving questions back to the student, see Chapter 3.) Expect to know less and less the longer you teach – and to feel happier and more confident as a result. If you don't believe me, ask some elder teachers.

Remember that, as yoga teacher Lizzie Lasater says:

Completing a 200-hour teacher training programme does not make you a yoga teacher. It is little more than an invitation to begin to learn how to teach yoga. It is an early step in a lifelong journey.[3]

You have many years in front of you to develop and hone your teaching. For now, enjoy being a beginner, exploring your new craft with a beginner's mind. There's no rush and no pressure.

REFLECTION

- What do you feel is the purpose of a yoga teacher? What are they meant to do?

- What do you feel is the nature of the relationship between yoga teacher and yoga student? What actions and attitudes on the part of the teacher can foster this relationship, and what actions and attitudes can stand in its way?

- Who are you as a yoga teacher currently? Is this who you want to be? If not, where are the incongruities and how might you begin to shift them?

- What are your intentions when you teach yoga currently? Are these a fit with your deepest, truest sense of purpose? If not, how might you begin to bring intention and purpose into alignment?

- How do you respond when a student asks a question you can't answer? What feelings does this bring up? Let your body inform you through sensations, images, feelings and (if you're lucky) spontaneous moments of awareness. Do any memories arise? Are there ways you could respond more skilfully when you don't know?

Apprenticing and assisting

If you feel unready to teach independently, one way to develop skills, experiment and make mistakes without carrying the full weight of responsibility for a class is to apprentice with or assist an experienced teacher. It's possible to get *loads* of support, information and free training out of this.

Choose a teacher whose style of practice and approach to teaching are in alignment with your own, and make sure that what they're offering is a match with what you're looking for. For some teachers, a teaching assistant is someone who puts out the mats and takes the money. Other teachers will create opportunities for their assistants to do some supervised teaching and will offer feedback and mentoring.

Assisting works best if you already have an established relationship with the teacher. If you're thinking about approaching someone who isn't your long-term teacher, do their classes regularly for a while before you ask. You are most likely to be taken on if you have demonstrated commitment and it can be seen in your practice that you understand how your chosen teacher works. Experienced teachers want assistants whose style and approach is compatible with their own because otherwise neither party can really offer much to the other. Anna, an experienced teacher who takes on assistants regularly, comments:

> Often, the email I receive from people wanting to assist is clearly a blanket one sent to many local teachers, and little thought appears to have been given as to whether we might be a good fit. For example, I was approached by one new teacher who teaches power yoga/ashtanga. I teach hatha. She said what she loved most was physically adjusting people to go deep. I rarely touch people at all, and when I do it's very light. I immediately felt that it wouldn't work. It depends a lot on how you reach out to existing teachers. Bear in mind that they probably get a large volume of requests for help and don't have the resources to help everyone. Be discerning in who you contact.

An added bonus of being an assistant or apprentice is visibility. Becoming known as a teacher in your local area is a priceless source of students and of offers of classes. You may also be asked to cover classes for the regular teacher, or they may pass on work to you that they are not able to take on themselves.

There's a lot more about apprenticing and assisting in Chapter 9.

Entering the community of teachers

My own teacher always said, 'There is a yoga teacher for everyone. That teacher may not be me, but that's okay.' And he is right.

Oliver

When I first started teaching, I was, as far as I'm aware, pretty much the only ashtanga vinyasa teacher in South East London, definitely the only one in Greenwich (the previous only-one had just stopped teaching to have a baby), and one of just a handful of yoga teachers of any sort in the immediate area. In terms of building classes, my primary task was explaining to people (1) what yoga was all about, (2) how ashtanga vinyasa fitted into this and (3) why they might want to try it. Yoga wasn't a normal thing that anyone might do, and there wasn't an existing body of local ashtanga practitioners; I had to cultivate it. Since then, the number of both yoga students and, to a greater extent, yoga teachers has exploded, and it's a very different landscape out there. The main problem for most new training course graduates nowadays is being seen in the jostling throng of teachers.

The majority of established teachers really want to welcome, help and support our new colleagues. Be aware, though, that from our point of view, there is an ongoing deluge of newly trained teachers onto the scene. While some of these have practised for many years and are genuinely engaged in offering yoga practices of substance which they have themselves embodied… others are not. Believe me, we have seen it all, heard it all, and most of us have been on the receiving end of unethical and unprofessional behaviour from new teachers, so forgive us if we are sometimes a bit jaded. Actions speak, and if you demonstrate that you are sincere in your desire to teach well, you will find that, on the whole, the established teachers in your area will get on your side.

Bear in mind, too, that an experienced teacher, known in their local area, is called upon to offer a lot of advice and support to a lot of different people. We all have finite amounts of time and energy, and it's necessary and healthy to set boundaries with regard to how much of it we can offer for no fee. While most experienced teachers are able to help a bit and answer some simple questions, there's a point where mentoring has to become a paid-for service or one of exchange. Remember that a senior teacher is not a free support resource for every new graduate in the neighbourhood; be reasonable and considerate in what you ask for, and you may well receive some help (see Chapter 8, 'Dealing with requests for free advice').

There are a few simple things you can do to step into your new professional field with awareness and have the best possible chance of engaging the good feeling and encouragement of your new colleagues:

- Make contact with the existing teachers in your area. Go to their classes. Make relationships where you can. See what you might be able to offer each other.

- Join any local professional communities for yoga teachers. Most areas have these, but if yours doesn't, you might want to think about setting one up, perhaps together with one or two other teachers. In my view, you are likely to get more from participating in yoga teacher communities if you do so primarily with the aim of making connections and sharing experiences, and only secondarily in order to market your classes.

- Avoid scheduling directly on top of an established yoga class (see 'Scheduling' below).

- Charge the going rate. Undercutting local teachers will make you very unpopular very quickly (see 'Pricing' below).

- Honour the groundwork that long-serving teachers have done to create an awareness of yoga, places to practise and interest in practising in your local area. It wasn't glamorous, and it probably wasn't lucrative.

- Respect the body of experience held by the senior teachers in your area. Find out more about what kind of class everyone teaches and any specialisms they have. This is going to be a resource for you when you encounter a student with an injury, health condition or other issue that you cannot competently include in your own classes.

- Be seen to be behaving ethically at all times – with concern for your students, with consideration for your colleagues, with attention to your own well-being, and with regard for the reputation of yoga teaching as a profession.

Obstruction from established teachers

One established local teacher whose classes I used to attend asked me to stop coming when she found out I was training to teach. The stated reason was that she was writing a book and didn't want me to know her new sequences!

David

It all turned ugly with my teacher when I was invited to teach an evening class at the venue where she was teaching – though her classes are only during the day. I asked her blessing, but she accused me of wanting to steal her students. I work part-time in a deli, and she told me, 'Stick to cheese. It's what you're good at'!

Agnes

It may come as a shock to realise that yoga teachers aren't all beautiful rainbow beings full of love and light. Some freshly minted teacher training graduates are quite naive about what they can expect in their new field of work. Be aware that the full range of human behaviours can be found among yoga teachers. While many established teachers will be, if not supportive, then at least too busy teaching to take much notice of you, there are those who will take down your fliers, bad-mouth you to potential employers, move in on your classes (scheduling an identical class on top of yours), and generally do their damnedest to cut you out of the market. It's not usual, but it does happen. As you would with any role, it's best to step into your new profession with blinkers off. Be realistic. Evaluate people's responses to you against commonly accepted standards. Be humble and considerate of others, but take your place with dignity, and don't allow yourself to be fleeced.

Don't hide your light under a bushel

I know that I need to promote my classes to be successful, but I'm nervous about advertising in case I upset any existing local teachers. I think I'm bringing something a bit different, but I'm aware that I'm the new kid on the block. Where is the line? How do I promote myself without stepping on the toes of established teachers?

Zoe

In order to make a class a success, we have to get behind our own offering and believe in our capacity to bring something of value. This is confidence – not hubris – and like other skills and capacities necessary for a yoga teacher, it usually has to be cultivated. We can be confident while still acknowledging our current shortfalls and deficits, and holding the intention to learn and grow. Every yoga teacher was once a beginner, and none of us was instantly skilled and effective. The challenges you are facing as a new teacher have all been experienced by tens of thousands of yoga teachers starting out in their teaching life. These are the experiences that build our capacity and enable us to hold more and more broadly.

It's perfectly normal and ethical to create classes and advertise them in your local area, and no established teacher can reasonably be offended by a new teacher doing this. Do your research to make sure that you are pricing in line with the going rate for your area and that you are not scheduling a very similar class over an established one. (See 'Pricing' and 'Scheduling' below.)

In order to thrive, a teaching and practising community needs an in-flow of new teachers. If you enter the community with an intention to support a healthy ecology, on the whole you are likely to seed classes and enterprises that flourish and grow, and that contribute to the diversity and sustainability of your environment as a whole. Teachers who operate in this way are generally welcomed and loved by both colleagues and students. There's no absolute guarantee against difficult or protectionist behaviour from some rogue established teachers (or even groups of teachers), but over time it's those who seek to nurture individual students, the local yoga community and the practice of yoga itself who become valued and respected teachers.

Self-employment and tax

As a yoga teacher, you will almost certainly be self-employed. If you have only ever been in employment before, this may feel daunting, but it's easy to register with HM Revenue & Customs (HMRC), and pretty simple to do all the record-keeping required to comply with tax regulations. I'm not an expert on any of these matters, but luckily yoga teacher/therapist and director of Yoga Tax Jessica Garbett is. Jessica has a tremendous amount of knowledge about the business aspects of setting up as a yoga teacher and has created a comprehensive series of free fact sheets on the subject, which are informative and easy to understand.[4]

Professional insurance

There's no legal requirement to have professional insurance as a yoga teacher, and the reality is that you're highly unlikely ever to need to make a claim. Nevertheless, it is generally considered best practice to insure yourself, and many venues and employers will require this. If you belong to a professional organisation (such as the British Wheel of Yoga, Independent Yoga Network or Yoga Alliance Professionals), insurance may be part of your membership package. However, you can also buy insurance independently. There are lots of providers and rates are competitive. I'm not an expert on insurance, so it's over to Jessica again for good, comprehensive information on general insurances.[5]

Professional organisations

While there's no requirement to belong to any professional organisation as a yoga teacher, in my view it is good practice. If you are a teacher who cares about the welfare of your students and takes your professional responsibilities seriously, you are going to want to be signed up and accountable to a professional body with a code of ethics. For your students this means that:

- They know you have met certain mimimum standards of training and/or experience.

- They know you are signed up to a code of professional ethics.

- If they have a complaint against you, they have an avenue to seek redress.

For you it means that:

- You have representation if a student makes a complaint against you.

- You have representation in the wider world – for example, a professional body will speak on behalf of its members if there are issues regarding legislation of yoga teaching, or terms and conditions of employment.

- You have somewhere to go for support and advice if you are treated unfairly at work – for example, by a studio that refuses to pay you.

- You may have greater credibility in the eyes of students and potential employers.

If you have completed a teacher training course, it will almost certainly be registered with a professional body, and on graduation you will be able to register with this body as a teacher. If you have come up in the traditional way – through practice, independent study and apprenticeship – and have no formal teaching qualification, it's possible to register with the Independent Yoga Network (IYN) via their 'independent training and experience' route.[6]

Be aware that not all professional bodies are made equal. While some are oriented towards service and representation, and may have not-for-profit status, others are more commercial in their outlook, or may be politically ambitious. Before you join any professional organisation, it's wise to ask existing members whether they have found it to be helpful, ethical and worth the membership fee.

Be aware, too, that no professional body regulates yoga in the UK, although some of them might like to give the impression that they do. There is, at the time of writing, no legal regulation of yoga here. You don't need training to teach yoga. You don't need teaching experience to teach yoga. You don't even need to have practised yoga – ever – in order to teach yoga. And you don't need to belong to a professional registering body. *Namaskaram*, the publication of IYN, has a good article – 'Regulation: The facts' – on regulation of yoga in the UK.[7]

Cover teaching

I thought, 'Yoga's everywhere these days. People do yoga at home, at work, in gyms, never mind in actual yoga studios. It's going to be easy to get work.' I couldn't have been more wrong. It's six months since I qualified. How do I get a chance to teach yoga?

Cherie

It's easy to get the impression from advertorial and social media that once trained, you have only to saunter into a yoga studio in a pair of designer yoga pants (in this context, something you put on *over* your knickers) and you'll be hired. Trainings, too, sometimes paint a rather rosy picture of your employment prospects as a yoga teacher. It can be a shock to find out how difficult it actually is to get a foot in the door.

Many teachers get their first break through cover teaching – teaching in the place of a teacher who is sick, on holiday or otherwise absent. Being the substitute isn't easy. You will be standing up in front of a group of people who would probably rather have their regular teacher and may need winning over. On the other hand, cover teaching is a great way to gain a wide range of experience and get exposure. It's often the cover teacher who gets the first offer of a class if the regular teacher wants to give it up, so covering can also be a route to permanent work.

The key qualities of a good cover teacher are availability, reliability and the capacity to teach to the style of the regular teacher. If you're blessed with the life situation to do so, being able to say 'yes' most of the time will guarantee you more cover offers. Don't run yourself ragged (a real danger – be mindful), but oblige if you can. At this stage, most work is good experience, and you will be able to refine what, where and who you choose to teach later. Make sure you know what type of yoga the regular teacher offers. No two teachers teach in exactly the same way, but you do need to give a class that is broadly in line with the students' expectations; that is, if you are covering a gentle hatha class, don't go in there with vinyasa flow. Agreeing to cover a class and not turning up – or cancelling at the last minute – is a capital offence in the yoga teacher rule book. If you let one teacher down, others will soon hear about it, and so will studio managers and gym class coordinators. It's hard to recover your reputation once you are known for being unreliable.

Ways to get cover work

- Contact gyms and yoga studios and ask to be added to their cover list. Usually, the person you need to talk to is the class coordinator (gym) or owner (small studio). The bigger, more established yoga studios are generally looking for cover teachers with several years of teaching experience already under their belt, but many gyms and smaller studios will take new graduates. Big chains usually have an application form; you will need a CV for small, independent outfits. You are most likely to get a result if you pop into the gym or studio and have a chat with the person in charge of the cover list. This way they will have a face for your name and will know that you are friendly and personable. Studio owner Joanie says:

  > If you regularly come to classes, we know you, the students know you, and you are part of our community, we are much more likely to give you cover work. We rarely add random people to the cover list.

- Go to the classes of local independent teachers whose style is similar to your own. Get to know them and tell them that you are interested in cover work. Don't do this the first time you meet them. Make a relationship first and let the teacher see that you are reliable and that you understand and appreciate the way they teach. It's a big deal to entrust your class to someone else – most of us don't do it lightly – so demonstrate that you are worthy of the responsibility.

- There are several very active and fast-moving yoga teacher cover groups on Facebook, such as Cover Me Yoga UK. Cover work is also frequently offered on Facebook groups for teachers in particular local areas – where I work ours is Yoga Teachers South East London. There may also be an email cover group in your area – ask around among other local teachers.

Making clear cover arrangements

I covered quite a few classes for a teacher who I thought was my friend. After several months of asking to be paid, finally I received a payment equivalent to £6 per class!

Domenica

Misunderstandings over arrangements for cover are very common. Often these arise because there is a pre-existing relationship between the two teachers concerned, and it is presumed that making a clear and comprehensive written agreement is not necessary. It is. The only time there's ever been a falling-out in one of my mentor groups was over a cover arrangement:

Teacher A asked Teacher B to cover a class without stating what the pay would be. Teacher B agreed to cover without asking about the rate of pay. A day before the class was due to happen, Teacher A informed Teacher B that the rate was £15 for the class. Teacher B withdrew from the cover arrangment because the rate was too low. Teacher A felt that they had been left high and dry; Teacher B felt that they were being offered well under the going rate and taken advantage of.

All of this could have been avoided if both parties had discussed the details and made a simple written agreement at the outset. Details you need to clarify in a cover arrangement include:

- How much the cover teacher will be paid.

- When the cover teacher will be paid.

- By whom the cover teacher will be paid – by the regular teacher or by the gym/studio/company which normally pays the regular teacher (see below).

- How much notice must be given if the cover teacher wants to withdraw from the arrangement.

Fees and payment

If you are covering a class for which the regular teacher receives a flat fee (in a gym or studio), you will normally be paid all of that fee. You can be paid either by the teacher or by the organisation that employs them. If you are covering in a big gym chain, you will need to be on their payroll. This is a bit of a faff and complicates your tax affairs if you are otherwise self-employed, but the advantage is that once you are on the books, you may be asked by the gym to cover other classes, and you can work at other gyms in the chain too.

If you're covering a class that the regular teacher runs themselves, there are a couple of fee options:

- The teacher pays you a flat fee. Pros and cons: There is no financial risk to you – bear in mind that in a teacher-led set-up, some students see covered classes as an opportunity for a week off, and you may end up with quite a small class. However, if the class is large, you won't see all the profit.

- The teacher deducts room hire and pays you the net profit. Pros and cons: If the class is busy, you stand to make more money – but if it's quiet, you may come away with not much, or even nothing.

However and by whomever you are paid, you will need to invoice them. An invoice should include:

- Your name and contact details.

- The date of invoicing.

- The date, time and place of the class you covered.

- The amount due.

- Your account details.

- Your terms (e.g. 'Please settle this invoice within 28 days').

- Your Unique Tax Reference (UTR) number.

Cover teaching etiquette

Never, under any circumstances, criticise the regular teacher or their teaching in front of their students. If you don't approve of what or how the teacher appears to have been teaching, bear in mind that all teaching arises out of a context, and when extrapolated from this, it can be difficult to understand. Remember, too, that what students report their teacher as having said may only mildly resemble what they actually did say! If students are doing a posture differently from how you prefer to teach it, try saying something along the lines of:

That's one way to work with this posture. Another way I like to approach it is…[explain what and why]. Let's see what happens if we try this approach today.

Different gyms, studios and independent teachers will have different views about what is acceptable in terms of cover teachers publicising their own classes. Some see the opportunity to acquire a new student or two as part of the remuneration package; others absolutely do not. Check the parameters in advance. On the whole, if a student asks you where else you teach, it's fine to give them details (it would be weird not to). Beyond that, be guided by the wishes of whoever is employing you.

Auditions

It's a little demeaning in some ways, don't you think? In what other field are qualified professionals asked to audition? 'We need a new pilot for our jumbo jet. Could you just fly this one to LAX so we can audition you for your flying abilities?'

Gideon Reeve[8]

It's not surprising that the 'audition' word raises the hackles of many yoga teachers. Teaching yoga is a relationship, not a performance. I first heard of yoga teachers 'auditioning' for classes around the time that yoga became a staple offering in gyms. 'Audition' wasn't a misnomer either. If you're unlucky enough to try out with an employer who expects you to twinkle and entertain, they probably don't know much about yoga, and you may want to consider whether this is someone you want to work for. A good employer will be more interested in authenticity, skill and your capacity to connect with and respond to students. Studio owner Franklin says:

> We both audition and interview potential new teachers. We want to see that the teacher has the skills and qualities we're looking for as a studio. We're responsible for ensuring good teaching standards for our students, so this is important. We also want teachers who are good communicators, are reliable and are focused on creating a sense of community. However brilliant and charismatic a teacher is, we will not employ them if they don't know how to work collaboratively as part of a team.

Being fairly old, I've only once been asked to audition for new work. It was a strange request, because I'd already been teaching weekly classes and running workshops for the organisation for about 10 years. I explained that I don't do auditions, but am always happy for someone to come and observe a class if they're not clear how I teach. No one came to observe, and I got the job. However, I was, at the time, an experienced teacher with an established reputation. A new teacher doesn't have this leverage, and if they want employment (rather than solely to run their own classes), they may have to negotiate the yoga teacher audition.

I asked some teachers (and one studio owner) for their advice on how to approach auditions. Here's what they suggested:

Be creative with your flow, without showing off. Give good verbal cues while making sure no one's getting lost or likely to injure themselves. (Aaron)

Be yourself. You may or may not be what they're after, but if you try too hard to be something you're not, you'll trip up. (Tanveer)

As a studio owner, I look for passion, warmth and individuality. I have to feel that the teacher would fit well in my studio and with our ethos, i.e., laid-back and down-to-earth. (Zena)

Teach authentically, from the heart. Make sure you get there early and give yourself time to ground yourself. (Mouna)

Show that you can think on the spot, keeping in mind the necessary protocols, such as correcting alignment, awareness of injuries, and a rhythmic and progressive sequence if you're teaching a flow form. Above all, just do what you do, to the best of your ability. (Talia)

Be sure to ask about injuries and health conditions. Gyms tend to be hot on that kind of thing. If you offer adjustments, ask permission first. Otherwise, be yourself, teach from your heart and try to enjoy the experience. You may find yourself in a group of instructors from different disciplines and be expected to participate in other forms of exercise as the 'student' as well as teaching them yoga. For one gym chain audition, I did two hours of zumba, circuit training, HIIT [high-intensity interval training] and core conditioning, and taught about 20 minutes of yoga. Personally, I found it a great opportunity to get a free work-out, try new things, meet new people and help others in the fitness industry get work. It was a long, hot, sweaty afternoon though! (Linda)

Speak clearly. If using music, don't make it too loud. Be confident, be yourself and enjoy it. (Dan)

Auditions are often about personality. You get 10 minutes to give a flavour of who you are. It's understood that you can't show every side of your teaching in that time. Choose a sequence you are comfortable with, and in which you can show your creativity. Hold the space as you would if you were teaching a full class. Be yourself and teach as you would normally teach. Be supportive of other people auditioning. Take part in their audition and use it as an opportunity to learn. (Thomas)

Notice a theme there? Yup. Number one tip: be authentic, be yourself!

Working in gyms

When I started yoga, back in the eighties, classes happened in church halls and community spaces. The fitness industry didn't exist, and gyms were few and far between and highly unlikely to offer yoga. These days, the gym is where many people first encounter and regularly practise yoga, and where a lot of yoga teachers get their initial opportunity to teach professionally.

Gyms and the sensory environment

In my observation (as an autistic person who works with others with neuro-divergence), a higher than average number of yoga teachers are autistic, neurodivergent or highly sensitive. If you are one of these teachers, working in a gym may be, for you, as for me, challenging, or impossible. Fluorescent lighting, pumping music, video screens and too many people in too little space add up to an environment highly conducive to sensory overload – one in which it is difficult to think, speak or process information. If this is your own personal experience, it's good to recognise and respect it. Though lots of yoga teachers do get started by working in gyms, it's by no means obligatory to begin here, and fine to stick to teaching in studios or creating your own classes from the get-go (see 'Working in yoga studios' and 'Setting up your own classes' below).

Be savvy

Many is the teacher who has been ripped off by a gym. While some gyms are excellent, dependable employers, others are fly-by-night, barely solvent and out to take eager new teachers for a ride. Don't be so desperate to get a foot on the ladder that you abandon all discrimination. Use the same common sense and require the same contractual agreements for a yoga job that you would for any other. Employers of yoga teachers are not inherently nicer or more ethical than the rest of humanity.

Fees and getting paid

The law of supply and demand has had a drastic effect on gym pay for yoga teachers. When yoga first entered the fitness industry, it was considered a specialism, and teachers were in relatively short supply. When I last did gym cover work, in around 2005, the going rate was £35/hour in London, with the more upmarket gyms paying £45, and one budget chain £25. A teacher with longevity in the job would generally be receiving a bit more. Nowadays, there is an over-supply of new 200-hour graduates on the market, some of whom would teach for nothing to gain experience, and the average fee in London is more like £25/hour – a drop of about 30 per cent, and that's without adjusting for inflation. Gym-based teachers have to teach *a lot* of classes to make a basic income.[9]

If you're teaching for a big chain of gyms, it often takes a while to get everything sorted out with the accounts department, and you can expect some initial glitches. However, once everything is set up and payments start rolling, the process is generally problem-free. Different gyms offer different payment terms. Some are fairly prompt, but others pay a couple of months in arears (you invoice at the end of the month, and the gym pays you at the end of the following month).

If you don't get paid

For the past four months I've been teaching in a new independent gym. Payment is due on the last Friday of every month. All the paperwork has been done, but so far I haven't been paid at all. I don't have a contract, just the invoices I have submitted. I've chased it up, but still no money. I have now heard that other teachers have not been paid either.

Mike

If you have not received payment within the expected time frame, and you have chased the payment with the accounts department, it's time to take some action. Threatening legal involvement may be all it takes to trigger prompt payment. Leanne says:

I was owed about £600 by one gym. I called the accounts department and told them that I had an appointment with my solicitor that afternoon. The payment was in my account on the same day.

If threats don't work, for a small fee you can make a claim through the small claims court. This is easy to do and can be initiated online. Make sure you go via the government service rather than through a third party (which will charge you).[10]

Pointers for working in gyms

On the whole, I have always run my own classes and have limited experience of gym yoga teaching, so I asked some teachers who are mostly gym-based what they would like new teachers to know about working in the fitness industry. These are some of their responses:

Hourly rates can be fairly low, but the work is regular, and you'll get paid the same even if there are only two people in the class (although if you're regularly getting only two, prepare for your class to be axed when the timetable gets reviewed!). (Lena)

Meet students where they are. Some people at gyms may just want to work on their flexibility, and that's fine. Don't evangelise the other aspects of yoga, but sneak them in when you can! (David)

Perks often include free access to facilities and classes. Find out what the gym is offering. (Alex)

Students in my gym classes tend to be in a very different head space from those in the classes I run myself. They may be distracted or just following along while looking out the window. I feel more as if I'm giving a performance in the gym. That said, there are those who want to learn, and the gym can be an entry point for going deeper. (Mary)

One of the main advantages of gym teaching is that the business side of things is taken care of. You don't have to do any promotion. The lighting, heating and air conditioning are usually good, and most gyms have a good selection of equipment, which means you don't have to lumber around with yours. I like the fact you get people who don't normally come to a yoga class – a much wider range of abilities and ethnicities. Some go, but some stay and become regulars. Disadvantages: the pay is crap. The classes are only a hour at the most – difficult to fit a well-rounded yoga practice in. New people are always dropping in, so it's difficult to build up continuity; you constantly have to start at the beginning again. You never know who's going to come through the door – but that's also what makes it fun and challenging. It's noisy: there's always music coming from the gym or other studios. People often wander in during the class, even though there's a sign on the door asking them not to. Most of the time, they just want some equipment or they realise their mistake, apologise and walk out, but sometimes they come in to talk to me – WTF?! (Paul)

You learn some great skills from working in gyms. Teaching multiple level classes is a given, as you never know who's going to walk through the door. You have to be able to modify for injuries (lower back, hamstring and shoulder being the ones I mostly come across), and you have to be able to break a pose down and build it up, offering variations for different abilities. Then there's the skill of helping students to find 'yoga' in an environment that's not really set up for it. Gym teaching has been an invaluable experience for me. (Joanne)

Get on well with the class coordinator. Attend a few classes (not just yoga) to be seen in the club and to get your face known. Coordinators love this. Always be on time for your classes and finish on time. Even if you're a great teacher, unreliability will lose you your class. Encourage students to be yoga sluts and try lots of other teachers' classes. (Sheila)

Gyms are regular work. The pay isn't great, but it gives a steady income. Things to be aware of: gyms can close down, be refurbished (so no classes for a while) or change hands (meaning a change of contract) all at short notice. Be prepared for any of these things to happen. (Andy)

I teach three classes a week in gyms. We have bricks, blocks and belts, as the members put pressure on the management to buy them. I mainly teach the same people every week: a very dedicated bunch, open to all sorts of practices including yoga nidra and meditation. Many of the gym members come to workshops I run, and that compensates for the pay which is generally £30 per hour. It's not a lot, but I don't want to work evenings, and gym classes can be the easiest way to have daytime classes. It really depends on who runs the studios as to how you are treated. In my gym we're lucky. (Marcia)

Working in yoga studios

How to be hired by a yoga studio? First, TAKE CLASSES AT THE STUDIO. Get a feel for the studio, the community, the teachers. Don't show up intending to get a job. Enjoy the class.

Second, TAKE ANOTHER CLASS THERE. Try a different teacher. Maybe the owner if you're feeling fancy.

Third, TAKE ANOTHER CLASS. Let the teacher and/or owner get to know you.

Okay, so now you think you're ready to try to get a job there? Then maybe chat to the owner about the fact that you are a teacher. Ask to join the sub list. Ask if they might be interested in auditioning you to see if you might be a good fit, because you may well not be. No offence. It's just fact.

DO NOT:

- *Ring up a studio you've never attended and say you're looking to teach locally and wonder if they're hiring.*
- *Bad-mouth other studios.*
- *Ask what style they teach.*
- *Ask where exactly the studio is located.*
- *Show up inappropriately dressed for the class you're taking because you genuinely have no idea what you're walking into.*

This is what I deal with regularly as a studio owner. Regularly. Please be better then this.

Alissa

Fifteen years ago, I could probably have counted on my fingers the yoga studios in London. Not only are there more, many more, studios nowadays, but there are also more types of studio. Some of the oldest are associated with particular lineages or styles of yoga. The Iyengar Institute in Maida Vale, for example, was set up more than 30 years ago, and the Sivananda Centre in Putney has also been going a very long time. Then there are the established high-end, multi-style studios, such as Triyoga and The Life Centre (both now with several branches). Small independent studios are currently proliferating across the city, some of them in areas that, from a demographic point of view, would not previously have been seen as willing or able to support a yoga centre. Latest onto the scene are the commercial chains, which operate on a membership model more akin to the usual gym chain set-up than the traditional yoga studio one. Inspired by market opportunity rather than a mission to offer yoga, MoreYoga envisages that by 2022 it will have opened 100 studios in London.[11]

An aura of glamour always used to surround studio work. It was hard to gain an entrée, with lots of competition and most studios requiring a lot of teaching experience, so there was a certain amount of kudos attached to being a studio teacher. The original big names still require substantial experience and ideally a reputation (good one) that precedes you. Triyoga, for example, asks for a minimum of five years, but says that most of its teachers have between 10 and 20.[12] Not all studios are made equal, however; as I mentioned above, it's possible to get a foot in the door of the small independent studios and of the commercial chain ones straight from a teacher training course.

Much of what has already been said about teaching in gyms also applies to teaching in studios. Some additional things to be aware of include:

- Some small independent studios are highly ethical and run on yogic principles. Others, however, are not. Many is the entrepreneur who has set up a studio and is out to make a quick buck from the yoga bubble. Be discriminating in who you work for and on what terms. Like small independent gyms, some studios are barely solvent and have no scruples about employing teachers in the knowledge that they are highly unlikely ever to be paid. These are in the minority, but they exist.

- If you take on a new class and then go away for a month, don't be surprised if when you return it has been given to someone else. Building a class takes hard work and consistency. The studio owner will expect you to be willing to show up and involve yourself in making the class a success. If you know you're about to go away, stick to cover teaching until you're in a position to invest your energy in a regular class.

- While a few new teachers quickly find a following, for the majority it takes time to develop the skills and knowledge to become a good teacher – one whom students will want to return to. If you're in this phase of your development as a teacher, it can be less pressurising to stick to cover teaching and running your own classes for the time being. Sky says:

It's stressful working for a studio because you're always worrying about numbers. A yoga studio is a business and has to be profitable. My classes got moved around a lot to fit in with other teachers, and in the end they were all axed. In my independent classes, it doesn't matter to me if only two people show up, and six is a good number, but six isn't enough for the studio to turn a profit. Now I just cover for the studio. It's a lot less pressure.

- Does your local supermarket allow rival chains to advertise in their stores? No, of course not, and it's the same with yoga businesses. Don't use your studio class to publicise those you run independently. This is the cause of many disputes with studio owners and may lose you your class. Most studios have rules about what you can and can't do in this respect; if this is the case, they will be stated in your contract, so read and observe them. Isobel says of the studio she runs:

> Teachers are not allowed to market their business within mine. I am the one paying for the overheads: the premises, marketing, administration and the cost of paying teachers even when a class has not made a profit. In my studio the students are my clients, and the teachers have to accept that.

In general, don't:

- Collect students' emails.

- Give out your own fliers.

- Talk to students about a class you run outside the studio.

If an individual student explicitly asks you for details about where else you teach, it's usually fine to give them a business card or a website address – if you don't, they're going to Google it anyway. It's a good idea to let the studio owner know that the student requested this information, just to make sure they don't get the wrong end of the stick.

Setting up your own classes

If you're self-starting by nature and prefer to be your own boss and do your own thing, you're probably going to want to run your own classes. One of the advantages of organising classes yourself is that you will tend to build a community of students who regard you as their teacher and come back week after week – which means that you can do much deeper work and that supportive relationships can form around the class. (This does sometimes happen with gym and studio classes, but it's less usual.) With your own class, you can be as experimental as you like, and you don't have to supply the kind of content stipulated by a studio manager or generate the number of bums on mats that a gym will require. If you prefer to offer a lot of individual attention, you can cap your class at six mats. If you want to make your class accessible to people without much money, you can set concessionary rates and offer work exchanges. Basically, you can set things up in any way that works for you and serves your own particular intentions.

A teacher who organises their own classes is also running a small business, and if this is an anathema to you, you may be better off sticking to working as a contractor (for gyms, studios, or anywhere else where the class is organised and marketed by someone else). Just as teaching is a practice, so – if approached with an intention of awareness – can running an effective and ethical business be. You are guaranteed challenges and opportunities for learning and growth on many levels.

Some of the key areas where you will require skills include:

- Administration – responding to enquiries, invoicing, contracting, record-keeping.

- Marketing – social media activity, designing fliers and posters, writing copy, maintaining a website.

- Finance – budgeting, pricing, keeping books, filing an annual return, making sure invoices have been paid, running a booking system.

While some yoga teachers have pre-existing business skills, many do not and learn on the job. It's worth finding out whether there is an enterprise board or other small business agency in your local area. These offer support, training, advice and other services to small businesses. It's usually free or low-cost. My first ever website was professionally designed, absolutely free, by Greenwich Enterprise Board. You can also out-source any areas of work you particularly detest or are spectacularly bad at (or both). For example, I keep my own books but pay an accountant to draw up and submit my accounts. Some teachers pay an admin person to do a few hours work a week for them or to deal with enquiries about a big event, such as a retreat or training course. Other teachers pay for the services of web designers or marketing professionals.

Venues

Good room space is expensive – especially in big cities – and hard to come by. Expect to have to look around and think creatively about how you might be able to use the space available. For example, a very small room could work well for a semi-private class (four people book for a block and pay something between one-to-one and group class rates); a cheap and cheerful space in a low-income area may be fine for a reduced-cost community class; a noisy venue could work for a high-energy class to music, with the teacher miked up.

When choosing and contracting with a venue, these are some of the key things you need to think about:

- Is the venue manager collaborative and eager to accommodate you? If they are, a less-than-perfect venue can often be made workable. If they really don't seem to care – or are plain obstructive – it may be better to look elsewhere, rather than wasting a lot of energy building a class that quickly becomes homeless.

- What's the heating like? Don't take it on trust that the room is lovely and warm in winter. If it isn't winter when you visit the space, ask other people who use it what it's like in cold weather. If you're teaching early in the morning or late in the evening, check what time the heating comes on and goes off. If the heating is just a bit under par, ask if you can bring in some electric heaters – but bear in mind that while these can give the temperature a boost, they won't have much impact on a chronically frigid room (high ceilings, drafty windows, ancient boiler, etc.).

- How quiet is the room? Community spaces are generally well used, and it's normal to expect some noise from other groups. While there's an obvious downside to this, being a part of a hub of community, among people of all ages doing everything from Cubs to capoeira, can be heart-warming and add to the class experience. For years, I taught a weekly led ashtanga class with the Greenwich Morris Men stomping away in their very clonky shoes and banging their very hefty sticks on our ceiling. Morris dancing became a standing joke in the class, and we managed to take it in our stride, mostly. Noise I couldn't work with in other venues was African drumming, and a youth theatre class with amped sound. I literally could not be heard over either of these groups.

- Is there safe storage space where you can leave mats and equipment? Or is there equipment at the venue that you can borrow?

- How do you and your students access the space? Will you be given a key, and if so, will you need to let students in? Is there a reception desk? When is it open and is it always staffed?

- Will you need to do any additional preparation before you use the space? Community venues are used for all sorts of things, and it's not unusual to have to sweep the floor and have a general tidy round before your class. Dance spaces are generally cleaner, with street shoes often banned from studios.

- How many mats can you *actually* fit in the space? If you're considering renting a yoga studio, you will probably have been given a mat capacity. Be aware that these sometimes err on the optimistic side(!), and may be feasible only if you're willing to have the mats more or less touching.

- Does the room hire rate include VAT or will this be added on top? Community venues usually (but not always) include VAT in the quoted rate, but dance studios and more commercial venues tend to add it on. Make sure you check before you commit.

- Is any get-in/get-out time included in your room hire or do you need to pay extra for this? Some venues include a standard 15 minutes either side of each booking, but others book classes back to back.

- What is the venue's cancellation policy? Are you required to pay for a whole term whether you're there every week or not? If you can cancel individual classes, how much notice do you need to give?

- Do you need to pay a deposit?

- Will you be invoiced in advance or in arrears, and what are the payment terms?

Make sure you have a clear written agreement with your venue covering all the bases, even if this is just in an email. This way you both know where you stand, and hopefully any disputes can be avoided.

Pricing

My biggest bugbear? New teachers cutting prices to a ridiculous degree in order to get people into their classes.

Gabriel

Do charge the going rate for a yoga class in your area – even if you feel that as a new teacher you cannot offer your students what more experienced teachers are able to provide. Undercutting existing teachers will not go down well and may mean that you lose out on support and friendship from your colleagues. Bear in mind that yoga teaching is not on the whole a lucrative profession, and many teachers are struggling to survive financially. Driving prices down is a race to the bottom in which it is the small independent teachers (not the chains of gyms and commercial yoga studios) that go under. These are often the people holding out for inclusion of *all* the many aspects of yoga in their teaching, who are working in unique, innovative and highly creative ways, and are concerned with offering meaning and an authentic experience to their students.

Just to clarify, we're not talking here about teachers bringing low-cost yoga to specific disadvantaged groups (people with mental health issues, migrants, carers, and so on); we're talking about the newly qualified teacher who sets up a general class, open to all, and charges £7 when the going rate locally is £12. If your intention is to serve disadvantaged groups, it's a good idea to ring-fence your offering, so that your class does actually consist of your target group – otherwise your student population can quickly become those who love a bargain and have spotted a cheap yoga option. One way to do this is to work with a charity in your chosen area. Another way to include people on a low income is to offer concessionary rates in your regular classes. This helps to ensure economic diversity and enables the more financially privileged to subsidise those who are less so, which is often appreciated by everyone in the class.

Teaching for free

There are situations where it's appropriate to offer your services for no charge, but if you feel called to do this, make sure it's for sound reasons. The yoga world is not short on teachers who lack a solid sense of self-worth, struggle to keep two feet on the ground and are slowly vitiated by ill-advised gestures of charity. Reciprocity is important for human beings. In order to serve both teacher and participants, a yoga class has to be constituted of a balanced exchange of energy. This is part of the holding of the class and is a kind of yoga class rule of physics. When that exchange isn't there, the structure can't hold, and people get hurt in the process of collapse. In our society, money most usually expresses the energy we exchange for a service, but we can exchange other things. An unemployed student, for example, might exchange some work in your garden for yoga classes. Students who really value yoga teaching generally feel more comfortable and are more willing to come to a class when they are able to offer something back. When no return at all is made, the teaching is often neither appreciated nor respected. It usually works better to invite poorer students to pay what they can afford or to pay in kind, rather than just waiving the fee.

Fee policy

Writing a fee policy can help you to clarify for yourself what your financial objectives are: what you are offering your students, how you are making your teaching available to those on a low income (if you are), and what you want to receive from your students in return. This is my fee policy:

> For most classes, there are two basic rates, one for those on a low income, and one for those on a medium and above income. There is also a financial hardship rate for people who are on a very low income who would not otherwise be able to afford classes. I ask you to be responsible for paying the appropriate fee. I don't do any checks. Take this as a part of your practice – it is! Please take into account your circumstances. If you're a retired person with two pensions and your own home, or a student supported by a well-paid partner, you're probably not in financial hardship. You may be if you're supporting other people and on a low wage. Please be aware that:

> - Classes and events have to be financially viable in order to take place.
> - The giving and receiving of teaching, therapy and facilitation is grounded in a balanced exchange of energies.
> - This work is the way I make my living.
> - Among the ethical foundations of yoga are *satya*, 'honesty', and *asteya*, 'taking only what we are entitled to'.

> If you can realistically pay the full rate, please pay it. If you need a lower-cost class, then please take one; it's of more benefit to me to have you at the class paying a small amount than not to have you there at all!

If you can't afford to pay anything, it's sometimes possible to arrange a work exchange. In this case I would ask you to make a commitment to the class and to the work. Please contact me to discuss if this is your situation.

Scheduling

The teacher who trained me always taught that when setting up classes we should look around locally to see what was already available, with a view to serving the widest possible student group, but also with the aim of respecting other teachers. She taught us always to ask ourselves whether we were stepping on anyone else's toes – and that if we were worried we might be, then we probably were.

Denise

Being mindful of what's already on offer around you when you schedule new classes serves everybody's best interests. Even if you don't care about professional ethics (and if you're reading this book, you probably do), scheduling a class in direct competition to one that's already established makes no business sense. You're far more likely to make money if you look for gaps you can fill.

What constitutes a gap is going to depend on any specialisms you have, the setting in which you teach, how dense the population is, and how many yoga teachers are in your area. Community venues in London, where I teach, are often supporting many yoga classes, and it would be ludicrous for a teacher offering vinyasa flow on Monday nights to get aerated about a teacher starting a new power yoga class in the same space on Thursday nights. On the other hand, I'd be very upset if another Mysore shala popped up in either of the two venues where Greenwich + Woolwich Mysore lives, or indeed in Greenwich or Woolwich. Mysore teaching is specialist work, our two rooms are well established, and there are plenty of other local areas with no Mysore practice at all: put your shala there!

If you are at all in doubt about whether your planned class will conflict with a pre-existing one, contact the teacher and check it out with them. Even if you know what you are planning will appeal to a completely different group of students, it's still considerate and courteous to talk to the other teacher and explain what your intentions are so that they are clear that you're not trying to move in on their territory. If they know a bit about the style you're offering and how you teach, they may even refer students who are better suited to your class. If you want to work in a culture of communication and collaboration, help to create it.

If you do inadvertently schedule a new class on top of an existing one, apologise and find a new time or venue. Don't grovel or put yourself down. Just acknowledge a professional error and make it good. Most teachers will be impressed by your concern for ethics, and you may gain a friend.

Student history forms

I was shocked to discover from a recent thread in an online yoga teacher support group that some teachers feel they do not have a responsibility to ask their students about health conditions and injuries. Apart from the possibility that not doing so will invalidate your professional insurance,[13] as yoga teachers we have a duty of care to our students. In order to be able to teach our students in the best way possible, we need to have a full picture of their body's history, as well as of any whole-person traumas, disorders or differences that affect them.

I recommend writing your own student history form. The PAR-Q (or Physical Activity Readiness Questionnaire) used by fitness professionals and lots of yoga teachers offers a good starting point but doesn't cover many aspects of health and history that yoga teachers need to know about, for example, mental health conditions, hypermobility and eye conditions that contraindicate inversion. You are probably also going to want to gear your form to the demographic that tends to come to your classes, so if you work with a lot of older people, you will need to ask about osteoporosis, arthritis, high blood pressure, and so on; if you teach trauma-sensitive classes, you will want more information about symptoms relating to post-traumatic stress disorder (PTSD) and developmental trauma; if your student group is mostly very active young people, questions about sports injuries and possible pregnancy are going to be relevant. It's also good practice to invite students to tell you about any particular needs they may have – and to do your best to accommodate these wherever possible.

You are likely to get a fuller response from a new student if you give them a written form to fill in and also talk to them about their general health and history. New students often don't understand what we need to know and why (even when it's explained on the form), and those who have been managing chronic conditions for a long time may just forget to mention what they live with every day. Don't expect students to disclose everything on first meeting.

Teaching is a relational activity, and relationships develop over time. See the form as the opening of a conversation that will continue for as long as the two of you are working together.

How we respond to any health or history disclosure a student makes is also important. I cannot tell you how many strange and unhelpful reactions I have received to disclosures of Ehlers-Danlos over the years. For example (and I didn't make these up):

What's that? Oh, hypermobility. You must be really good at yoga!

What's that? Oh, hypermobility. You must find yoga really easy!

I'm very flexible too. My knees do this [demonstrates weird knee thing]. My shoulders dislocate a lot as well [pops them out of joint]. I find the splits really easy [drops into a spaghetti version of *hanumanasana*].

And to my mind, the most invidious (this one from a senior and high-profile teacher):

That's just a story.

Generally, the most useful way to receive any information your student gives you about their health and well-being is to listen and ask a few basic questions:

- How does that affect you day-to-day?

- Are you aware of any movements that make the pain better or worse?

- Has the specialist told you to avoid any particular kinds of movement?

- Is there anything I can do or not do to enable you to participate more fully?

Anyone can be wrong-footed. If you respond in a way that you realise is inappropriate, apologise and start again. The person will most likely forgive you and will probably think all the better of you for admitting a mistake. If you've never heard of the student's condition, be honest; don't try to blag it:

I haven't come across POTS. Can you tell me a little bit about what it is and how it might affect you during the class?

Remember that the person with the condition is always the expert on how it affects them – but don't interrogate them or expect them to educate you about their condition. Go away and research. If you do this consistently, in tandem with working in collaboration with your student, you will gradually build up a body of practical knowledge about how to accommodate a wide range of health conditions and differences in a class.

'I know how to work with it'

When a student discloses a health issue, they often add, 'but I know how to work with it'. If they're an experienced practitioner, this may well be true; however, it's not really the point. When we seek student information as teachers, it's so that *we* 'know how to work with it'. It's important not to be deterred from seeking the detail you need in order to include the student in the class safely. For example:

Student: I have a knee problem, but I know how to work with it.

Teacher: Tell me a bit more about the knee problem.

Student: My left knee tends to 'wobble' a lot. I can't do half-lotus position.

Teacher: Have you had the problem diagnosed by a physio or orthopaedist?

Student: A physio diagnosed it, but I can't remember what she said it was.

Teacher: Was it damage to the cruciate ligaments? If they're torn or over-stretched, your knee will usually feel unstable. They sometimes get injured in an impact trauma where there's twisting.

Student: Yes, that's it. I tore a ligament in a skiing accident a few years ago. It's a lot better but it has never totally got back to normal.

Teacher: That's fine. We can look at how you support your knee when we do postures involving external rotation. You can tell me what works, and I may be able to suggest some things you haven't tried before.

In my experience, 'I know how to work with it' can be a cover for a range of different meanings. Sometimes it's a defensive response to past interventions by teachers who were not knowledgeable about the person's condition or collaborative in working with it. In this case, it's important to acknowledge the student's authority over their own body, to express your willingness to work together with them, and to convey – honestly – your own competence to work with their condition. (If you don't feel competent to work with it, say so and either refer them to another teacher – if you think they are not safe in your class – or tell them you don't know much about the condition, but will do some research and hope to learn more about it through working with them.) 'I know how to work with it' can also mean, 'I won't take up too much of your time and energy' or 'Please allow me in your class – I can cope'.

In this case, the person is likely to feel reassured by your willingness to spend time talking to them at the outset, and offering variations, modifications and technical tips during the practice. In either case the real question is about your capacity to hold the person in practice. When your response suggests that you create a kind and secure class container, they are likely to relax and work readily with you.

Legal waivers

On many teacher trainings, the student history form is presented together with the legal waiver as one document; however, these are actually two separate entities. Personally, I don't ask students to sign a waiver: I don't want to set up my relationship with them on a legalistic basis. In any case, no one can sign away their legal protection. In the rather unlikely event that you are taken to court by a student, it's by the law that the case will be judged, not by what the student put their name to on a waiver. I do, however, include a statement of responsibility on my class joining form. This currently goes:

> While on the whole yoga practice is beneficial, some postures are contra-indicated for particular health conditions, as are some physical adjustments, so I need full and up-to-date health information in order to work with you safely and appropriately. Your details will be kept confidential and shared only with assistant teachers. You are responsible for disclosing all relevant information and keeping me updated about any changes.
>
> Yoga can involve some physical adjustment of the body. If you don't want to be touched, that's fine. Please let me know in advance of the class.
>
> We will be working carefully to minimise the possibility of injury. However, please be aware that yoga can be a physically challenging practice. You are responsible for respecting your own limits and staying within them.

Teaching full-time

> When I gave up my PAYE [pay-as-you-earn] job to teach yoga, I moved into a shared house to minimise my outgoings. I teach 14 classes a week, which involves a lot of travel. I also teach a few one-to-ones, which are a bit better paid, but my income is still very low. I don't want to live communally forever. I feel like giving it all up and getting a normal job again.
>
> Angela

I make very little profit by the standards of our society. But when I look at my annual accounts, a lot of my business expenses relate to yoga events, travel and trainings that were great fun and enormously fulfilling. I don't have much disposable income but my lifestyle is amazing, and that for me is far more important than money.

Margot

If you pay any attention to social media, you could be forgiven for viewing yoga teaching as a glamorous job, characterised by sun-kissed beaches and designer leisure wear. The reality is that teaching yoga is mentally and physically demanding, and sometimes quite stressful. One hour of contact time may require many more of preparation, adminstration and marketing. And if you thought your daily commute was tedious, bear in mind that many yoga teachers have to make multiple long and time-consuming journeys every day in order to clock up enough classes to make a basic income. For a new teacher, who is likely to have to take classes when and where they can get them, and who will probably need to do more than the usual amount of preparation, the actual job is likely to be even further removed from the fantasy one.

To make it as a yoga teacher, by and large you have to be:

- A talented teacher – or a marketable one.

- Determined to teach, no matter what.

A tiny number of superstar teachers make a very good living from yoga, but on the whole, yoga teaching is not lucrative. The majority of us get by on a very modest income and with little or no financial security. If big holidays, nice clothes and fine living are important to you, don't become a full-time yoga teacher – unless you have financial support from a well-paid partner or savings from a previous well-paid job, own your own home and need only a small top-up income from teaching yoga.

Consolidation

If you're a new teacher aspiring to teach full-time, you may well have accepted every yoga job you've been offered – in every style of yoga you can conceivably teach, in every area you can possibly manage to travel to, and often for very poor rates of pay. Your schedule will probably have you zigzagging across town like an ant on acid, hanging around for two hours in the middle of nowhere until your next class and then rushing frantically to make it in time for the start of class number three. It may be hard to find time to eat a meal and do your own practice, and you may not have a regular day off every week, never mind the glorious two that most employed people take for granted.

In the longer term, this way of life is obviously not sustainable. In order to teach full-time and be happy and healthy, you need to create a sensible schedule, one that hangs together and gives you a decent basic wage. This entails emptying your rag bag of classes, looking at what you've got, giving away what isn't usable, and considering how the rest might be stitched into a useful and harmonious garment. This is a process; it takes a bit of manoeuvring and requires some persistence.

Some aims and objectives include:

- Shifting all classes in one geographical area to the same day or days. This will entail some ducking and diving and requires patience: waiting for venue space to open up, for a gym to revise its timetable, for a teacher to be willing to swap classes, and so on. Make it known to gym coordinators, studio owners, venue managers and local teachers that you would like to move a class. All of this can feel like the Rubik's® Cube that never quite gets solved, but keep at it, and gradually things will click into a more workable design.

- Specialising. Classes for pregnancy, back pain, cancer, and so on give you niche skills and access to a different market. Think about which student groups you have a particular affinity with and which kinds of work interest you. See if you can assist a teacher already specialising in this area so that you can find out what the work is really like and get some practical experience before you invest in training. Once you're qualified, let other local teachers know about your specialism so that they can refer to you if they need to.

- Creating an independent class to slot into any empty spaces in your day. This is where specialisms can come in handy. If you have an early morning class and a lunchtime one, for example, you could fill the mid-morning with a chair yoga class in a care home, a carer and baby yoga class or some yoga teaching in a school.

- Deciding when you want to teach and focusing all your energy there. For example, if you teach a lot of early morning classes, don't take on any more evening work and begin to lose or swap out the evening classes you already have. You may prefer to work only in the evening or (like me) only in the daytime. This kind of ring-fencing is do-able over the long term, and important for your well-being and longevity as a teacher. You need to eat, sleep and generally have downtime.

- Picking two days for your time off and beginning to move or let go of teaching work on them. You can have your 'weekend' whenever you like (mine is currently Thursday/Friday), but make sure you have one, and make sure the two days are consecutive. It takes time to wind down and relax properly.

- Looking for higher-paying work. If all your work is in gyms and small studios at £25 per class, you are going to need to do an awful lot of teaching to make a basic income. One-to-one sessions and workplace classes are much better paid. Retreat teaching is another option.

Maintaining your own practice

I used to love my yoga practice and would get on my mat every day, no problem. Since I started teaching, though, I'm finding it hard to do my own yoga. I've taken on a lot of gym and cover work, and by the time I get onto my own mat, I'm feeling tired, uninspired, and reluctant to do yoga. I really miss the old joy and enthusiasm.

Stephanie

The rite of passage from yoga student to yoga teacher often involves a shift in relationship with our own practice. When I first started to teach, I felt that I had been given licence to get on my mat. Yoga was now legitimately at the centre of my life, and I no longer had to justify the large amount of time I spent engaged with it. On the other hand, as a new teacher it's common to find it difficult to maintain a previous practice. What you once did regularly may seem too challenging or just too long to fit into your schedule. Yoga may no longer feel like a fun thing you do just for yourself; there may be pressure to perform; and if you're teaching a lot, by the time you get onto your own mat you may just be fed up to the back teeth with yoga.

Personal practice often starts to unravel when we are imposing an unrealistic idea about what we 'should' be doing upon the actuality of what is needful and practical in our circumstances. It's important to keep in mind that you are not in service to your practice; your practice is in service to you. If practising doesn't feel like a resource and a nourishment, something is out of kilter. Frame your practice as an open and inviolable space. You can use it to dance, rest on a bolster, draw, write a poem or move through an ashtanga vinyasa series. Any activity that conduces to embodiment is welcome here. Your practice time is for you, so don't use it to try out sequences for classes or do other teaching preparation. This is time for putting something back in, not more giving out.

When our personal practice is deeply and thorough-goingly self-oriented, it also becomes the compost for our teaching, not because we are thinking about themes for classes or considering how best to articulate the structure of a posture in words, but because we are feeding our own roots as a practitioner. When we have this vitality of own practice, we can teach out of the exuberance of our own growth. We don't have to regurgitate what we once long ago discovered but which no longer has life for us, or what others have taught us, because we are in a daily process of emerging our own enquiry. As our yoga practice segues into our teaching practice, we also engage our students in this ongoing investigation, so that between us we generate a field of embodied curiosity that expands and enriches the experience of everyone in our practice community.

REFLECTION

- What is your current practice like? Has it remained constant or has it changed in any way since you became a yoga teacher? If so, how?

- How does your current practice serve you? Are there ways in which it does not serve you? If so, how might it change to be more supportive of your present needs?

- What is the relationship between your personal practice and your teaching practice? Is it a healthy one? If not, what may need to shift?

EXPERIENTIAL WORK: MOVING INTO THE FIELD

This piece of work is an exploration of how you are entering the field of your new profession. Entering is a movement, so movement will be the medium here. When we work experientially, witnessing ourselves is like sitting on a river bank watching the river. The water may be fast, slow, powerful, turbulent, torrential, rippling, burbling, babbling...but it's never wrong. It's just the particularity of one river in one moment in time. So it is when we observe the river of our own being. You can't be right...and you can't be wrong.

You can do this exploration alone; it can also be powerful to work with one or two other new teachers and to witness each other.

You will need:

- Paper and a pen for writing, or materials for drawing.

- A clock, watch or timer.

- Optional: music and something to play it through.

- At least 30 minutes of undisturbed time in a private space where there is room to move. You can take a lot longer if you like.

1. Decide how long you're going to move for. Ten minutes is about the minimum, but you could dance for 90 minutes or more. Just make sure you choose a length of time that you will definitely be able to commit to.

2. Sit quietly for five minutes or so and reflect on your entry into the profession of teaching yoga...then let your reflections dissolve.

3. Now for the movement. Begin however you need to begin. Your body may hurl you immediately into motion...or you may need to lie quietly on the floor for a few moments first, allowing movements slowly to emerge. Your movement may be a dance, or it may be something stranger and more mysterious, more like play or like clowning, or like nothing you've ever seen before. The intention is not to perform your thoughts, ideas and feelings about becoming a yoga teacher - these are things you already know - but to allow movement to arise spontaneously. You are looking to emerge information you have not until now been aware of.

4. Allow the movement to follow its own trajectories and let these be surprising. As much as you can, avoid editing or censoring - but if you do edit or censor, mark this for yourself, without making it wrong. This is just another useful piece of information. If sounds emerge, allow these through: voicing is also movement. Be committed to staying in movement for the duration of the time you've set yourself, even if your movement is tiny (fingers fluttering) or repetitive (jogging on the spot). If it's hard to keep moving, notice that, without judgement. If you get bored, notice that, without judgement. All experience is grist to the mill.

5. When your moving time is up, sit down with your paper and pen or drawing materials and reflect on what you noticed. You can write, scribble, doodle, draw, tear up your paper... Do whatever feeds the process of discovering, marking and integrating. Questions for reflection might include:

   i.   Was it easy to move? Did you move fluidly and readily? Was it difficult to move? Did you feel obstructed, weighed down, constrained...?

   ii. What was your movement quality? Brisk, staccato, energetic, stomping, joyous, timid, restrained, apologetic, graceful...?

   iii. Did any memories arise? What were they? Do any feelings go with the memories?

   iv. Did any emotions arise? Were these expected or surprising?

   v.   Did any images arise? Do any feelings go with the images? What happens if you stay with some of the images and allow them to lead you in writing or drawing?

   vi. Does your experience of moving resonate with your experience of becoming a yoga teacher? Where are the similarities? Where are the differences? Is there any new information here?

Working with others

If you're working with a colleague or colleagues, each person moves, one at a time, while the others quietly witness. When everyone has moved, all of you transition into the reflection process and do this all at the same time, solo.

You may want to introduce these additional steps.

1. After each person has completed the set time for their solo moving, join them on the floor and move with them for a period of time. You could work out in advance how long this will be or you could just move together until you sense that the dance has reached completion.

2. When you have finished the period of reflection in writing or drawing, take five minutes each to share with the others anything you would like about your experience in movement. The others listen without commenting. Make sure this doesn't become a conversation: one speaks; the others silently witness.

3. If you are a group of experienced witnesses and are able to reflect in words on what you see in another's movement without projection, you could add another round in which you speak about what you observed as each person moved. Only do this if you are confident that everyone can own their own experience. This is advanced!

EXPERIENTIAL WORK: MISSION STATEMENT

For this exercise we are going to repurpose some business tools. You will be emerging your core values in your work as a yoga teacher and creating for yourself a mission statement. The intention is not to generate copy for your website or draft an element of a business plan (although the results of this exploration might form the basis for either of these) but to capture, for your own information, your key intentions as a teacher.

You will need:

- ◉ A pen and paper.

- ◉ At least 45 minutes of quiet, uninterrupted time, but you can take longer if you like.

1. Follow the instructions for 'Entering the terrain of your body' in Chapter 1. It's important not to leave this step out, otherwise you may embark on the exploration wearing a business head, and that isn't the intention.

2. Pick up your pen. You are going to write for five minutes, without pausing, about what really matters to you in your teaching. Why did you decide to teach yoga? What gives you most satisfaction? When do you feel that you have done a really good job? What makes you get up off the sofa and head out to a community hall at 6pm on a Thursday night? Be sure to include thoughts that come from left-field, that you aren't sure about or that you don't understand. If you get stuck, keep writing 'stuck, stuck...' until things start flowing again. Notice anything you want to edit out and, if possible, include it. No one is going to read your writing except for you, unless you choose to share it.

3. Read through what you have written, looking for the essential underlying values. Each value should be a single word or phrase, and you can have as many as you like. Your values will be unique to you, but to give you an idea, some might be:

    i. Embodiment.

    ii. Joy.

    iii. Service.

    iv. Creativity.

    v. Community.

    vi. Love.

    vii. Ethics.

    viii. Spirituality

    ix. Functional movement.

On a new piece of paper, write your values down in a list.

4. Pick up your pen once more. You are going to write for five minutes, without pausing, about who you really want to teach and why. Let your thinking be expansive. Keep writing. Don't stop.

5. Read through what you have written. Circle or underline the groups of people you feel particularly drawn to work with. On a new piece of paper, write your key groups down as a list. Your priorities will be your own, but might include:

    i. Elders.

    ii. Children with learning difficulties.

    iii. Ordinary people in my local area.

    iv. Prisoners.

    v. Professional dancers.

    vi. People with back pain.

    vii. People with cancer.

    viii. Athletes.

    ix. People who are really committed to yoga.

6. Pick up your pen once more. You are going to write for five minutes about your intentions as a yoga teacher. What do you really want

your students to receive? Don't worry if there is some overlap here with what you wrote for point 2. Don't edit. Don't stop. Think broad and deep.

7. Read through what you have written. Circle or underline any intentions that feel particularly important to you. On a new piece of paper, write these down in a list. Your intentions will be your own, but might include:

    i. To connect people with their bodies.

    ii. To offer simple embodied awareness practices.

    iii. To alleviate physical pain.

    iv. To offer techniques for transformation.

    v. To help people to live in a healthier and more mindful way.

    vi. To reach people who wouldn't otherwise have access to yoga.

8. Read through your values, your key student groups and your key intentions. These are your raw material. You are going to use them to write a short mission statement (maximum six sentences) about your work as a yoga teacher. This should express the essence of what you are here to do, why you want to do it, with whom and why it matters. Remember, the statement in this exploration is not for commercial purposes, so you can make it as off-the-wall as you like. You're not trying to sell anything. The point is to clarify for yourself what you're about as a yoga teacher when you get down to the nitty gritty.

Keep your finished mission statement and read it any time you feel unsure about your direction and in need of reconnecting with your core purpose.

3

Skills and Tools

In this chapter we will be looking at some of the teaching skills and tools that are less often articulated in teacher training courses but which are foundational for rich, meaningful and effective teaching. When we witness a seasoned teacher, there is often a sense that they are simply being themselves rather than doing something. Over the years, they have embodied their material so that it emanates from them; their teaching skills have become naturalised; and they have a sense of comfort with the teaching situation that allows them simply to inhabit it. While you may not yet be quite so accomplished, you can cultivate habits, approaches and tools that will grow your teaching practice in this direction.

Language

Language is a powerful teaching tool. The words we choose and the way we deliver them are significant components in creating spaces where our students feel nurtured, supported and encouraged to explore. Teaching is generally most effective and student-friendly when you speak in a way that feels native to you, and lots of different styles and idioms can work. However, there are a few general guidelines that may help you to communicate in the most skilful way possible.

Say what you want (not what you don't)

It's generally most effective to teach towards the positive, so if you intend for a student to draw their elbows into line with their shoulders in a headstand, say, 'Draw your elbows into line with your shoulders' rather than, 'Make sure your elbows don't go wider than your shoulders'. This doesn't mean that you should never, ever utter a negative. In dialogue with a student, for instance, when you are expanding on why it may help them to line up elbows and shoulders in their headstand, you might use many different ways of phrasing. But when you're issuing a simple instruction, say what you want to happen.

Affirmation

One of my long-time dance movement teachers peppers her facilitation with, 'Yes, just like that'. This is affirmation. The effect is to enable each individual in the group to settle into exactly what's happening for them in the moment, irrespective of whether it seems like what other individuals are doing or feeling. Sitting down quietly next to a student and whispering, 'Yes…good… yes…' as they slowly release into a tight spot, or telling your group, 'Exactly that…yes, everybody…' reassures, supports and encourages each person to trust their somatic experience and drop deeply into it.

Instruction/suggestion

A skilled yoga teacher is able to communicate shapes, forms and structures with clarity and precision…and to invite students into personal exploration of formless, somatic space. They also know where instruction is what's needed and where suggestion is appropriate. If we get this wrong in our facilitation, our students are going to feel confused (suggest, when you need to instruct) or frustrated and intruded upon (instruct, when you need to suggest). Foundational to yoga, and a capacity that we all want our students to have, is subtle internal attention. This 'feeling into' allows us to sense and respond to the needs of our own physiology. At the same time, a new student has no concept of the structure, appearance or intention of a posture. They can't inhabit it, because they don't know what 'it' is. So while we want to allow scope for feeling, receiving and adapting for the particularity of our own anatomy, we also have to give our students a clear template for each posture.

If you want a specific result – for example, everyone raises their right hand – you need to give a specific instruction. Don't use, 'you could', 'maybe' or 'if it feels right'. This doesn't communicate that you are articulating an element of the foundational architecture of the posture and that you need everyone to do what you are asking. For example, if I'm leading a beginner-level ashtanga class into *utthita trikonasana*, I might start by saying:

> Step your right foot forward, roughly one of your own leg-lengths... Turn
> your back toes slightly in and orient your hips towards the long side of your
> mat...letting the upper hip roll slightly forwards... Check that your front
> heel is lined up either with the heel or with the instep of your back foot...

The languaging of these instructions is clear, simple and precise. It avoids
words like 'perhaps', 'feel', 'explore' and 'see if'. These are all appropriate for
an experienced student who knows the form of *trikonasana* well and is in
an established practice relationship with it; they are not appropriate for new
students who want to know where to put their right foot.

If, on the other hand, you're leading a slow mindful class, in which the
intention is for each person to be guided by their own internal trajectory,
attention to interoceptive and somatic experience is the point of the practice
and standardised form is of little importance, you will want to avoid direction
and choose invitational and exploratory language instead. In this kind of
facilitation, there are lots of qualifiers, articulations of choice, and signage
towards individual, inner experience. For example, at the beginning of a
restorative yin yoga class I might say:

> Allow your attention to drop into your body and open your attention to any
> sensations you're aware of... If emotions...thoughts...images...memories...
> also arise...you may want to include these too... Know that at any point
> you have the choice to move towards a sensation...emotion...thought...
> feeling...memory...or to move away. You may want to notice the natural
> play of inclination towards...away...towards...away...

Even in this kind of class there are points at which structure is required.
Towards the end, for example, when students resurface from practice, explicit
instruction is needed to help them out of process and back into ordinary
consciousness, so that they are once again fully present and safe to go on
with their day:

> Begin to tune into the sounds around you... Notice your contact points with
> the floor... Be aware of yourself in the room, lying on the floor, in your body...

A clearly demarcated shift from suggestive to directive language in itself
signals to students that we are beginning to dissolve the practice container
and reorient awareness outwards. At this point we also need to make sure –
not take it on trust – that students really are once again capable of hearing
and following directions, and that they are fully back in the here and now.

REFLECTION

- Do you tend to teach through positives ('do this') or through negatives ('don't do that') or through a mixture of both? Have you noticed any differences in the results?

- Do you offer affirmation to your students? What kind of words and phrases do you use? Just enough affirmation, and a student feels seen and validated; too much, and they may feel patronised – how do you get the balance right?

- How do you use language to instruct students into postures? Does the language you choose match your intention? Is there language you might want to change? How might you change it?

- How do you use language to guide somatic process? Are there ways in which your language could be more open and less directive? Are there specific words and phrases you might want to adopt...or lose?

Make every word count

I've been working on eliminating 'just' from my teaching vocabulary for about 15 years; I've got better, but it's still a work in progress. There are, of course, many good uses for 'just', when it does the work of meaning in a sentence, but it's often an empty filler. For example:

Just allow your breath to settle back into your belly.
    Allow your breath to settle back into your belly.

Just take a step to the left.
    Take a step to the left.

Just let yourself just experience the sensations.
    Let yourself experience the sensations.

Unfortunately, I've now developed a 'so' problem:

So let's repeat this posture.
    Let's repeat this posture.

So if you find this too challenging...
    If you find this too challenging...

So just bring your hands together.

Noooooooooooo!

Most of us have certain favourite redundant words: 'kind of', 'actually', 'really', and so on. They often fill in when we feel unsure and unwilling to put our money where our mouth is, and they can quickly become habits of speech. We live in a culture in which women are trained to soften words, to be inoffensive and unassertive in speech; as a result, it can be especially difficult for female teachers to eliminate filler worlds. Having the capacity to come straight out with what we want to say, without mitigating it unnecessarily, can make a big impact on how we are seen as a teacher – how knowledgeable, confident, senior and experienced – and how seriously what we say is taken.

It may be helpful to record yourself teaching, notice where you use filler words, and practise saying the sentences without the excess wordage. This can feel surprisingly exposing. Notice any feelings that come up, and go gently. Remember, this is long-term developmental work.

REFLECTION

What are your most-used filler words? What effect do you think they have on your teaching? How would it feel to teach without using them at all?

When in doubt, shut up

When I'm observing new teachers at work, a piece of feedback I often give is: make room for silence. We live in a world stuffed to the brim with words – conversation, emails, text messages, advertising, public transport announcements... Most of us are starving for non-verbal spaces. As teachers, it's easy to feel that we have to to fill every second of our teaching time with explanations and instructions. We may be driven by the need to give our students their money's worth, or to prove that we know 'enough' to be standing up in front of a class. The reality is that silences are not a deficit but rather a positive addition to our offering to our students. Jason Crandell advises:

> Don't tell your students everything you know about each pose. Some teachers, your author included, are tempted to fill every second of each class with instruction, precaution, lore, personal revelation and more... Don't overcrowd your students or compete with yourself.[1]

How much we speak is, of course, going to depend a lot on the style of yoga we're teaching. Jason Crandell suggests sticking to 'an average of three instructions per pose'.[2] If I'm leading an ashtanga vinyasa class, in which I count everyone through the series, my role is a bit like conductor of the orchestra: I'm binding together a group of disparate individuals and maintaining the musical texture. If I stop speaking the numbers of the count, the names of the postures and the directions for accessing them, the practice will probably grind to a halt. What I can do, though, is create a sense of quiet and spaciousness by speaking sparely – without embellishing the basic instructions – and maintaining a measured pace and even tone. This doesn't mean I never give technical guidance, but that I'm judicious in how much and where.[3] It's like knitting a garment with loose tension rather than tight.

If you know that you tend to 'knit tight', it can be a helpful discipline to pause for a beat between sentences. For example, if you're leading a sun salutation:

Inhale: bring your arms up (pause for a beat).

Exhale: fold forwards (pause for a beat).

The beats here replicate the pauses within the breath cycle (for more on this, see the experiential work 'Breath' at the end of this chapter), and as such can help your students to feel how the movements they are making need not be random but can arise out of the natural expansion and contraction of their own breath. For some students, feeling this connection can be revelatory – and life-changing.

In a more static class, in which postures are held for a longer period of time, try counting slowly to 10 every time you feel the urge to speak. If you're teaching a yin or restorative style, you may want to extend the silent sections to three…or five…minutes. Use a timer if you need to. If you're a teacher who is always bursting to speak, *make* yourself keep schtum for all of the designated silent time. Notice any feelings, memories or associations that arise. You may want to note these down so that you can explore them in your own practice, or with a mentor or therapist.

Savasana

What really ruins savasana for me is a teacher who talks all the way through it.

Andrew

Savasana is essentially a silent practice. You will probably need to use language to help your students transition into and out of it, but when they are actually in *savasana* – don't talk! If your class is up to an hour in length, be sure to allow at least five minutes of silent time; if your class is longer, allow 10 minutes or more. By the way, don't use *savasana* as an opportunity to pop out for a break. Your students are still in practice; they still need you to hold the container; and for some, *savasana* is where the need of holding is greatest of all.

REFLECTION

- Do you allow sufficient silent time for your students to metabolise their experiences in your class? If not, what might be getting in the way? What might you need in order to be able to shut up a bit more?!

- Do you knit tight or loose when you are leading a sequence? How might it be to loosen your tension and include more silence?

Use your real voice

If you were a small child in the early seventies, you may remember Mr Benn.[4] Every week, wearing a bowler hat and black suit, Mr Benn left his house at 52 Festive Road for the fancy dress shop – and emerged from the magic door at the back of the changing room dressed as a knight or a fireman or a cowboy. For some of us, putting on our yoga teaching voice is a bit like that. It's a suit of armour that enables us to stow away our normal self and have a great adventure – as someone else. Kat Heagberg says:

> When I first started teaching…I was really concerned with not sounding yogic enough. I didn't want to be myself. I wanted to be a yoga teacher… I spoke with my yoga voice – a soft, lilting head-voice that I hoped sounded ethereal enough to drown out my awkwardness.[5]

What our students most want from us, though, is authenticity. You would think it should be the easiest thing in the world to show up and be yourself, but for many of us it's terrifying to sit in the teacher seat without the filter of performance – just sitting, just speaking, just being in relationship with our students and sharing what we know. All of this requires a willingness to be vulnerable that we may only acquire as we mature and gain confidence in teaching.

There are a few performed voices that crop up frequently in the yoga world. These are my top five (you may be able to come up with more of your own):

- Soft porn star: breathy, seductive – especially prevalent when the teacher is miked.

- Minstrel: sing-song, with odd, rolling musical phrasing, often hard to understand.

- Nursery nurse: overly care-takey, with use of baby language ('let's roll over onto our tummies').

- Cheerleader: excitable and overly encouraging ('Go for it!', 'You can do it!', 'I'm so proud of you') – more prevalent in endurance- and fitness-based approaches.

- Priest: intoning, paternalistic, authoritarian – most often adopted by revered and would-be revered senior teachers.

All of these voices contain a grain of something valuable: appreciation for the sensuality of the body in movement; the desire to nurture; knowledge and experience; the wish to encourage and support our students…however, they lack the breath of real life. They may be temporary rental voices tried on by a new teacher, or may have become habitual and fixed.

So how do we begin to ease into our real voice? Here are a few suggestions:

- Make it an intention to speak to your students in your normal voice at least once in every class. Not before or after the class, but during. Plant the seed; it will grow.

- Mark the voices that crop up in your teaching…and notice which feel real and authentic to you. Also notice any feelings or assumptions that go with each voice. This can be a powerful awareness practice. You don't have to do anything in response to what you notice (although you can if you want); awareness in itself is a great mover.

- Thank and formally release any voices you would like to let go of, acknowledging how they have helped you. For example:

    Bossy head girl, thank you for showing me how to hold strong boundaries in my teaching. I now release you.

- Pick one short section of the class, perhaps at the beginning or the end, and use it to practise speaking in the same tone of voice and idiom that you might with your family or friends.

- Look for places where it feels safe to be a bit more of yourself…and let yourself out.

This piece of work is essentially about expanding your comfort zone, which is something that has to happen *slowly*. If you exceed your actual capacity, you will trigger constriction, so accept the inevitable gradualness of the process. Be aware, too, that expansion and contraction are two phases of a single cycle; where we have expanded, we are bound afterwards to experience some contraction. Let's say, for example, you realise you become overly serious when you teach and decide to risk making a joke during your next class. Students laugh; all goes well – but afterwards you feel ashamed. The inner dialogue goes something like:

> Why did I say that? I made myself look so stupid. My students will never take me seriously again.

Relax. This type of response is totally normal and natural. Just notice your thoughts and feelings and don't take them too seriously. They come, they go. The more you practise bringing your own voice into your classes, the smaller the subsequent reactions will be, until, like waves in disturbed water, they level away.

In my experience, pretty much any authentic voice can be appropriate for teaching, as long as it's audible and comprehensible. You may be able to think of beloved teachers with eccentric vocal patterns, weird phrasing and strange modes of delivery that nevertheless really communicate. The key thing is that the voice intrinsically belongs to the speaker and that they fully inhabit it.

REFLECTION

- Do you use your real voice when you teach? If not, how might it feel to allow this voice into your teaching? Are there barriers you are aware of? How might you begin to approach these?

- Which voices emerge when you are teaching? What do they tell you about your intentions and values as a teacher? Are any of these voices excessive, over-used or performed?

- Are there teachers whose voice really works for you? What qualities does it bring to their teaching? What does it tell you about them, their intentions and their values as a teacher?

Keep your voice in the middle ground

Obviously, it's necessary to vary your tone somewhat according to the kind of class you're teaching. The voice required for an energetic power yoga sequence is going to be different from the one that serves in a yin yoga class. If you're teaching in a large room, you will need to project, whereas in a small room, normal speaking volume will usually suffice. That said, though, on the whole aim to stay expressive but pretty even – not monotonous, just even. As the teacher, you are holding the ground for your students, and the sound of your voice is part of how you do that. If your voice becomes over-excited when the energy in the group rises, you risk losing the guy ropes and ending up with over-stimulated students who struggle to settle at the end of the class. By the same token, if your voice becomes too flat when the group drops into a quiet passive posture, you will most likely hypnotise your students or lull them to sleep. Remember that your voice is part of the class container. It should be responsive to your students but not overly influenced by their experiences. You are the vessel, not the water.

REFLECTION

- How do you use your voice to hold the container for your students? Is there anything different you would like to try?

Give questions back to the student

I really value teachers who don't over-teach, don't spoon-feed students, let them make their own way, mistakes and all, not only to build skills but also to create resilience and responsibility. I try to constantly ask myself the question while teaching: 'Am I teaching them this for me and my "standards" or for them and their true development?'

Amy Hanlon (yoga teacher)[6]

As a teacher, you possess a body of knowledge and experience that many of your students do not yet have access to. Some of this you can share by telling your students, but much of it cannot be conveyed through instruction and narrative. Rather than trying to be an oracle, it's helpful to refer some questions back to the student for their own exploration. This underlines for them that while you can offer structure, support and some information, their practice is their own, and ultimately only they can answer their own questions. For example:

Student: What should I be feeling in this posture?

Teacher: I'm going to offer that question back to you. Notice what you're experiencing in your body. What kind of sensations and where? How intense is each sensation? Do any thoughts or emotions go with it? Take time to explore this for yourself and let me know what you find out.

Some students are very ready to give over their self-authority to the teacher, and this is not healthy. Some teachers believe that they are responsible for having all yoga-related knowledge at their fingertips and conveying it to their students – which is not healthy either. Shucking off some of your students' proffered questions allows the student to pick them up and try them on for themselves. This creates a sense of mutuality in a relationship that can very easily become verticalised.

Referring the question back is a great tactic not only with students who lack confidence in the authority of their own experience but also with those who are unboundaried in their requests for your time. These are the students who keep you hanging on for half an hour at the end of every class when you're tired and hungry and just want to go home, but they want to know what's going wrong with their jump-through; or the students who email rambling queries that only a small thesis could do justice to. A response in this situation might be:

These are complex and interesting questions. I invite you to take time to explore and investigate them. The real yoga happens when we start to emerge our own answers.

REFLECTION

- Do you do your best to answer all your students' questions? If so, do any feelings arise when you think about *not* answering some of them?

- If you're not already giving some questions back, where might there be opportunities to do this?

Slow down and honour the spaces

Integration is a whole-person experience involving not only the rational brain but also the nervous system. It takes time and (relatively) empty space. If you stuff your class with postures, techniques and information, students will quickly become over-stimulated and may leave feeling over-excited, angry, wired, hyper or ungrounded. This is a kind of energetic indigestion.

It requires some experience to feel into the appropriate pace for a class. Generally, new teachers tend to go too fast and try to pack too much in. If your own nervous system is agitated, as it may well be if you are a novice teacher (you feel nervous, terrified, tense, on edge, unsure, panicked), it becomes even harder to tune in, and the tendency is to follow the sympathetic response and speed up.

The desire to produce a smooth and seamless class surface can be another driver in the elimination of those empty spaces which are actually helpful resting places for our students. The antidote here lies in forestalling the impulse to plaster over the joins, allowing yourself to be fallible, in process, in the moment and on the wing, and your class to be imperfect. You cannot control the teaching process – and should not, because to do so mitigates against deeper and more organic learning opportunities for both you and your students. Try allowing natural pauses to stand when, for example, you:

- Choreograph a sequence.

- Reflect on an idea that has just occurred to you.

- Search for a word or a way to articulate a thought or form.

- Ponder which way to go next.

This applies to fast-flowing classes as well as to slow and relaxing ones. Indeed, my experience is that the faster the choreography, the more internal slowness and spaciousness is required in order to keep the whole thing calm, fluid and on the ground.

Many people are less able to process speech when they are focused intensely on their body, so your normal conversational speed is usually going to be too fast for facilitating movement. You can slow yourself down and make your speech more comprehensible by leaving spaces between words… phrases…and sentences. Pause to weigh your words and allow them to sink in. This will have the effect of aerating your class with little bubbles of space. It's also helpful to repeat key phrases slowly, calmly and evenly. Every teacher will have their own style; the words you choose, and the way you use them, will be unique to you. This is a way I might use pause and repetition in a led ashtanga class (with the counts for five breaths):

> *One*…as you fold forwards…allow your in-breath to expand…into the lower back ribs… *Two*…breathe into the lower back ribs…so that you are increasing the spaces between your back ribs…at the same time that the front body wraps in… *Three*…and lifts up and under the front ribcage… lifting up and in, right under the front ribcage… *Four*…so there is closure in the front… Expanding the back ribcage… *Five*…lifting, wrapping, closing beneath the front ribcage…

Don't use this many words for every *asana*; so much language will be overwhelming for your students. Just pick a few postures where you want to add more detail.

REFLECTION

- How do you honour the spaces in your teaching? Are there other ways of including spaces that you would like to try?

- Do any feelings arise when you contemplate allowing more spaces into your teaching? And when (if) you do actually allow those spaces in your teaching, are the feelings the same?

Touch

> *I teach a daytime class which is attended by quite a few older people. I like to give gentle hands-on assists – my students appreciate them. One elderly lady told me that the main reason she comes to the class is to receive the assists, because otherwise she would not be touched by anyone.*
>
> Hazel

As babies, we are literally touched into our skin – into an awareness of our individual body boundary and of the boundaries of another – and we go on needing to be touched all our lives. Touch is such a simple thing – and yet it isn't. Perhaps at no other time in history have those of us living in the Western world been so aware of, and so sensitised to, the prevalence of abusive touch. As a *Yoga Journal* article of February 2018 puts it:

> Rocked by #metoo stories of sexual misconduct in the yoga community and beyond, students, teachers, and organisations alike are speaking out – and figuring out where we go from here.[7]

Simultaneously, increased interest in and research into how trauma operates in human organisms has led to a better understanding of the role touch can sometimes play as a trauma trigger, resulting, in turn, in the development of no-touch approaches to yoga for those with PTSD and developmental trauma.

Touch can be sexual, violent or intimidating…and it can also be integrative, assistive, reassuring or just friendly. It can trigger trauma memories and it can also be a crucial aspect of recovery from trauma. It concerns me – a lot – that in the abuse scandal fall-out, touch itself is sometimes being pathologised, and outlawed from our yoga rooms.[8] Words, too, can be abusive, and can also be trauma triggers; do we therefore stop speaking to our students? Of course not. It's how we use words and with what intention that matters. The same is true of touch. It's healthy to include touch in relationship with your students – with awareness and respect for individual boundaries. As Melanie Cooper (yoga teacher and trainer with a specialism in adjustment) says, 'Human touch is healing and nurturing; it creates connection and resonance between the teacher and student.'[9] That yoga can expand our repertoire for, and our sensitivity to, touch as a form of communication is one of its great gifts. If anything, now is the time that we need touch in our yoga rooms more than ever before.

For more on touch see Chapter 4, 'The ethics of touch'.

Adjusting

When we talk about adjusting, what tends to arise in the popular yoga mind is an image of a teacher manipulating a student's body – often quite forcefully – into a particular predetermined shape. This is really the dark side of adjustment. I see adjusting as a form of body contact communication happening on multiple levels, some of them common-or-garden and immediately evident; others subtle, intuitive and difficult to capture in words. This is a capacious definition, and it includes a lot of possible intentions. The following are a few that feel important to me; you can probably add more of your own.

Holding the form

The adjuster provides the underpinning for the posture, holding its shape for the practitioner (as appropriate to the way it manifests in the practitioner's own unique body) so that the practitioner can feel into the form and begin to find the neurological pathways to create it for themselves.

Creating safety

Supportive touch can make a frightening place feel safe enough to enter. This kind of adjustment might be a hand behind the heart at the beginning of a drop-back to *urdhva dhanurasana*, or a finger on the sacrum in a challenging standing balance.

Showing where

The adjustment indicates where a muscle needs to activate, or breath needs to be directed, or the point of balance needs to shift. Whereas words require translation, touch is the direct language of the body. When the two systems, of teacher and practitioner, are tuned into each other, this kind of adjustment can be a powerful and transformative experience – a form of *shaktipat*.

Integration

I first learnt integrative touch, many years ago, in training as a Phoenix Rising yoga therapist. This kind of adjustment offers witnessing and (physically expressed) empathic presence, helping the nervous system of the student to settle and metabolise an experience, especially one that has been emotionally activating. This might be a hand on the sacrum in child's pose following a headstand that has aroused a lot of fear, or hands placed on the back in a counterposing forward fold when a student is over-excited after a strong back-bending sequence.

Shifting the structure

Where the fundamental set-up of a posture (often, but not always, a standing one) is out of kilter, a knowledgeable and sensitive adjustment may resolve the structure quickly and easily – whereas it might take a lot longer to achieve the same thing through words. This kind of adjustment is very useful in a busy and fast-moving gym or studio class containing students with little yoga experience. Check that the student is happy to be touched and make sure that they have an appropriate stance before you attempt to adjust: if you adjust the top on an unfeasible bottom, you will only end up with a different kind of skew-wiff.

Enabling

A little extra can help a student to achieve a posture and be a stepping stone to getting there on their own. We use this kind of adjustment a lot in the ashtanga vinyasa system, for example, to enable a practitioner to bind in *ardha baddha padma paschimottanasana* or *marichyasana C*, to drop back and stand up again from *urdhva dhanurasana*, or to pike into a handstand.

Stretching

Speaking as an oldish person with Ehlers-Danlos, I never want this kind of adjustment, but I teach people who really do and who get a lot of benefit out of attuned and biomechanically knowledgeable stretching. Use with care – be clear that you have the person's consent, and check in frequently as you adjust to make sure all is well.

Moving out of extremes

I often use adjustment to move a practitioner out of a situation in which they are focused on pulling one joint into end range of motion. The intention is to reconnect them with forgotten body parts and encourage them to work in a more balanced way. This kind of adjustment tends to create greater physical comfort and biomechanical functionality.

Permission to adjust

> *Should I ask permission before I adjust my students? We never did this in my teacher training, but at one studio where I teach, it's the policy to ask students before we touch them.*
>
> Coral

Gaining genuine consent to adjust is quite a complex process, involving unspoken negotiations with pre-existing expectations of what happens in a yoga class, the power balance between student and teacher, the set-up of the class, and so on. In a busy class, in which there is a constant traffic of new students, in my view it's good practice to ask students before you adjust: 'Would you like an adjustment here?' Students often assume that the purpose of the adjustment will be to push them 'deeper' into the posture, so it may be necessary to clarify:

It may help to change the way you're approaching the posture so that it feels a bit more comfortable for you and you can feel the shape we're aiming for a bit better.

It's important not to make the request be about something *you* want to do. I've also heard, 'Is it okay if I touch you?', which sounds a bit creepy. Remember, this is about something you can offer the student, if they'd like it.

In ashtanga vinyasa, which I mostly teach, there is a pre-existing expectation that the teaching will involve adjustment, so on the whole it's more of an opt-out system than an opt-in. On my website and on booking forms I include this statement:

> Ashtanga teaching includes some hands-on adjustment of the body. If this is not okay for you, please let me know by email or at the class.

If I'm teaching a led ashtanga class that includes students who are new to me, before we start to move I often say something like:

> The assistant teacher and I are going to be moving around the room helping you. If you particularly want to be adjusted in a posture, please attract our attention and we'll try to get to you. If you don't want an adjustment, that's completely fine. Just let us know. We won't be offended. This is information we need. Please also let us know if an adjustment isn't working for you or is too strong. We really want this kind of feedback so that we can work with you in a helpful way. We can get an idea of what's happening in your body by looking, feeling and sensing, but so far we haven't developed psychic skills and we don't know what you're experiencing, so please do communicate with us!

When I'm actually adjusting, I check in with the person frequently:

> How does this feel?

> Is your knee/shoulder/ankle okay?

> Is that about right, too much or not enough?

Be aware that a student saying they consent to an adjustment and the same student *actually* consenting to the adjustment are not necessarily the same thing. Students may be afraid of displeasing or offending you if they decline an adjustment, or (I put my hand up to this one) they may override their own sense of what's appropriate for their body because they want to experience the adjustment and are curious about where it might take the posture. If you are sensitive and attuned to your students, you will develop an embodied sense of whether you really have consent. This is an ongoing conversation. Keep listening and be alive to how things change. A student who usually loves adjustment may sometimes not want it, while the student who hasn't been up for adjustment before may come to trust you and want to dip a toe in the water.

Personally, I don't seek consent simply to touch (as opposed to to adjust), because for me touch is part of ordinary everyday human communication, and we don't usually ask permission to do that. Just as we mostly have a sense of when someone is or isn't willing to talk to us in words, so we usually know, if we're paying attention, whether or not they are willing to interact through touch. It's a given that we're going to get it wrong sometimes – and then, together with the other person, we negotiate the mistake. This is part of the normal to and fro of human interaction.

For more on the ethics of touch see Chapter 4.

REFLECTION

- Are you comfortable with giving and receiving touch? If not, what are the challenges for you? How do these show up in your teaching? Is there work you need to do? Skills you need to practise? Edges you need to approach? Would you benefit from some kind of support here?

- Do you use adjustment in your teaching? If so, what intentions do adjustments fulfil for you? If you don't yet adjust, are there any forms of adjustment you would like to experiment with? If so, how might you begin to introduce these into your teaching and where might you get any necessary training?

- How do you ensure safety when you are adjusting? How do you make sure that adjustments are as consensual as possible? Is there anything else you need to do in either of these areas?

Get off your mat

I took on several new and inexperienced teachers on trial when we opened. The teachers I've let go of are the ones who never leave their mat.

Giovanna (studio owner)

Teaching is about much more than standing up front and leading a sequence. In order to teach effectively, you need to interact with your students. To enable the average gym or studio group to embody the basic set-up of a posture, spoken direction, repetition, clarification, marking (showing key aspects of the posture) and individual adjustment are all going to be necessary. It sounds obvious, but when you're a new teacher and your mat feels like a little island of safety, it can be daunting to move out into the room and connect with the individuals in it.

One way to deal with this is to go cold turkey: don't have a mat. I sometimes don't bother with a mat when I'm teaching, or I fold it up and use it as a cushion for sitting. If you need to mark part of the practice, you can do that anywhere in the room, and you seldom need a mat to mark. If that sounds way too terrifying, commit to making a few forays into the water during every class you teach. You can move off your mat to:

- Witness the room from a different vantage point.

- Smile encouragingly at someone.

- Give verbal feedback to an individual student.

- Offer a simple adjustment.

- Reassure a student who appears anxious or out of their depth – humour often works well here.

There's an art to keeping the class in motion while you are off your mat and teaching individually. I have a more projected voice for the whole group and a much quieter, more intimate one for an individual I'm working with in the moment. The more you practise, the more skilled you will become at vocal multi-tasking.

REFLECTION

- Are you comfortable leaving your mat when you teach? If not, what gets in the way? Are there skills you need to develop? Fears you need to explore? What do you think might be the benefits of moving out into the room? Are there any downsides?

Teach without demonstrating

I'm feeling exhausted and am in a lot of pain. I teach 12 classes a week. They're all vinyasa flow, and the demonstrating is really killing me. I can't afford to drop any classes. What can I do?

Samira

Being an excellent teacher doesn't require the capacity to demonstrate. Indeed, preoccupation with demonstrating can get in the way of effective teaching.

In order to teach regularly and to have longevity as a teacher, it's essential to be able to work without doing all the postures yourself. For many people, making this shift is part of the passage from practitioner to teacher. When I work with new teaching assistants, I often initially ban demonstration. This compels them to develop the capacity to teach through voice and touch. Once they are skilled at teaching in this way, I allow them to mark particular aspects of a posture that they want to draw to the student's attention. A yoga class is – or should be – much more than a game of Monkey See, Monkey Do. We want people to be able to emerge the postures from their own body, rather than trying to imitate the way they appear on someone else's.

This way of working enables the teacher to spend most of their time watching and responding, and therefore particularly serves beginners, who really need our full attention. When we are preoccupied with doing postures, we are not available to offer much to our students. I have many times witnessed a new assistant teacher in our Mysore room moving through a posture with their back to a student, blissfully unaware that the student has lost the plot and ground to a halt, or is contorting themselves into the kind of shapes that would immediately raise a red flag if the teacher could see them. Letting go of demonstrating forces us to slow down and explain more – rather than overwhelming students with long strings of movements that they can't remember and haven't really understood or embodied.

It's often injury or burn-out that prompts the movement away from doing the postures and towards teaching them. If you are in this situation, know that you are not alone. Few and far between are the teachers who have never had to manage physical incapacity. It goes with the territory. Teaching with an injury presents a great opportunity to embody care for the injury and to articulate verbally the ways in which it is possible to stay in personal practice while physically less than one hundred per cent. This is a teaching that many students really need to receive.

On the whole, don't ask a student to stand at the front and demonstrate for you. For one thing, this is a waste of a great opportunity to invite all your students to step up and really embody (rather than simply copy) the postures. More invidiously, it sets up a hierarchical class dynamic, with those who are able to demonstrate (that is, produce a *Yoga Journal* cover version of the postures) at the apex, and everyone else trailing along somewhere behind. Value everyone's practice equally, whatever it looks like. Remember, too, that a student who is demonstrating is forfeiting their practice time – even if they are willing to be up front. Class time is – or should be – undisturbed space, hallowed ground, for giving attention to our own experience.

REFLECTION

▨ Do you feel confident teaching without doing the postures? If not, what stands in the way? Are there any learning edges here you need to meet or skills you need to acquire? Do any feelings arise when you think about teaching in this way? How do you imagine it might be?

Teach from a chair

I'm a big fan of teaching from a chair. I like the way it up-ends people's expectations of what happens in a yoga class – and in the space where the expected isn't happening, there's room for something new to arise. Sitting in the chair subverts the preconception that the teacher will be able to do all the postures perfectly and that the student's role is to copy the teacher. Shifting the emphasis away from follow-along reorients students towards listening, feeling and finding the unique expression of the posture in their own body.

Being a Mysore teacher, as I am, entails teaching for three hours at a stretch, often following a two-hour own practice. I also have Ehlers-Danlos and POTS (postural orthostatic tachycardia syndrome), so my capacity to stand is pretty limited. I started to include a chair in the Mysore room because I needed to sit down. I wanted to own my physical limits in a very visible way, and in so doing offer permission to my students to own theirs too. When possible, I now also have a chair if I'm teaching a led class. I get up and wander around all the the time to adjust and offer individual suggestions, and I sit on the floor a lot too, but I also return to the chair from time to time. It offers a unique perspective on what the students are up to, and it reminds me of what my role really is in the class.

You don't need to wait for a physical limitation (disability, injury, pregnancy) in order to explore teaching from a chair. The experience is available to you at any time. Give it a try. You will find you are enormously freed up to witness the class, and therefore to offer teaching points that are specific to the unique group of students in your room.

REFLECTION

■ How much physical energy are you investing in teaching? Does it feel sustainable? Are there alternatives you might want to explore. How might it feel to do less in classes? How might it feel to teach from a chair?

There is no 'peak' pose

Framing one posture as the 'peak' pose encourages students to strain towards it and tends to create a grasping mindset. Rather than teaching an apex posture followed by 'modifications', offer a platter of different variations. Present these horizontally, as equal but different expressions of a single posture, of which any one might be a better fit for an individual body. Let go of the hierarchy, and invite your students to be fully present to what their body is doing now, rather than leaning into attainment. This way of working will help to mitigate against injury in your class and will create a climate of equality, in which there are no 'advanced' students, but rather a community of uniquely skilled practitioners each approaching the same piece of work in a different way.

REFLECTION

■ How do you offer modifications to your students? Do some of your students tend to strain towards a 'peak' posture? Are there ways you might make your teaching less vertical and more horizontal?

Welcome emotions

The partner of one of my students died suddenly about a month ago. Today, she returned to the class for the first time. When we went into savasana, I saw that she was in tears. I decided it was best to let her cry – I had the sense that she needed this release. At the end of the class, the student came to talk to me, and afterwards we had a hug. This is the first time I've had an experience like this. Did I do the right thing? What do you do if someone cries in your class?

Elise

The body is an ancient storehouse of not only our own but also our ancestors' emotional experiences. These are stitched into our tissues – cells, organs, fascia, bones. Whatever we have been too scared, angry, young, overwhelmed or frozen to feel, the body holds, until we are ready to let feeling into consciousness and express and integrate it. One of the gifts of a somatic practice such as yoga is that it offers an opportunity to unpick old seams. When the time is right, a particular movement or a certain touch can send a thread unravelling out of time, releasing memories and emotions we did not know were there. This is a process of clearing and making space, as a result of which we are able to move forward a little less encumbered by the invisible baggage of the past, with a sense of being lighter, freer, more joyful and at peace.

We can expect our students to experience emotions in our classes. This isn't something going wrong: it's exactly what's meant to happen. As Rod Stryker says, 'If you have never laughed or cried in a yoga class, what are you waiting for?' As the teacher, our role is to include, witness and hold the student, with their feelings and the release, without shutting any of it down or making it wrong. We also need to frame what's happening in such a way that the rest of the group can be comfortable with it, and no one rushes in to 'comfort' the emotional student (which may put a lid on their process of release and integration). Every situation is slightly different. But in general these are some of the things I might do if a student is emotional in a class:

- Check in with the person briefly. Let them know that what's happening is completely fine and that they are in a safe place to allow it to happen. This may occur simply through a hand on their shoulder.

- If you think they might appreciate it, offer them a blanket or a gentle restorative posture where they can be with the feelings and allow them to move through in their own time.

- A student in an emotional state will sometimes want to leave. If you can, make it possible for them to stay in the room, include their experiences in the practice, and be included by the group. They will usually feel more able to stay if you defuse any sense of shame around showing emotion and normalise the experience of emotional release:

> It's really good that you're allowing these feelings to come through. Emotional release is something most of us experience from time to time when we're practising yoga. You are very welcome to be in the group, just as you are, and know that we are all supporting you as we continue our practice.

- Name what's happening for the rest of the class in a simple, straight-forward way:

> Ben is fine. He's taking some time out to feel some feelings. Let's support him by continuing our practice and giving him space to be however he needs.

- When you get to *savasana* and whatever closure you do at the end of the class, bring the person back into synch with the group. It's helpful for the welfare of the whole group to name that the person is okay and is joining back in with them:

> Ben, are you ready to sit with us? That's great. Let's come together and take a moment to honour all our different individual experiences during the class...and appreciate the support we each offer one another, just by being here, practising together.

This way everyone knows that their classmate isn't lost in distress, but has negotiated their experience and returned to the group. Witnessing this process can be powerful for some students. Formally rejoining also helps the person who has had the release to transition back to normality and be ready to leave the room and go home.

- After the class has finished, check in with the person. If they want to tell you something about what they experienced, listen, receive and affirm. Don't give advice or offer opinions. If they don't want to say anything, let it be. Make sure that they're in a state to negotiate the outside world and get home safely.

If a student is still very distressed at the end of the class and seems unable to move through their experience, it's likely that they are encountering some significant trauma and would benefit from professional help. A Phoenix Rising yoga therapist, Somatic Experiencing practitioner or body-centred psychotherapist would be a good referral. Alarm bells should sound if a student repeatedly goes through the same emotional process in your class without any resolution: they may be retriggering, rather than processing, trauma. In this case, you might want to suggest to the student that they get professional help before they return to the class. Be clear that this is because you are concerned that doing the class is reinforcing an unhelpful trauma response – not because their feelings are unwelcome in your class.

Crying is just one form that emotional release can take. It's quite common for people to giggle. Another response might be a burst of rage. Sudden feelings of dizziness, heat or cold can also be somatic responses to the expression of a held emotion. The student may or may not have a sense of what has been released. Some held experiences date from before we had language or the capacity to make sense of what was happening to us. It isn't necessary to have a memory or an explanation in order for a held emotion to be processed. Encourage your students to accept what has happened as an ordinary helpful event that doesn't need analysis.

REFLECTION

▨ Have you experienced emotional release in your own practice? How did you feel afterwards? Have you ever had an emotional release in a class? How did the teacher include it and make it welcome? Is there anything they could have done differently?

▨ What kind of emotional release responses have you experienced among your students? How did you include these experiences and make them welcome? How did this work? Is there anything you might do differently next time?

Be yourself – judiciously

Be yourself, be authentic: it's axiomatic for yoga teaching, and for good reason. Teaching under an assumed identity is neither engaging for our students nor satisfying for ourselves. As Kat Heagberg says:

> If you're teaching from a place of authenticity, it's going to resonate with your students. I know that when I shifted my aim from being 'perfect' to being authentic, teaching became a lot less stressful, a lot more fun, and way more sustainable.[10]

However, there is a small but important caveat here. Good teaching entails being yourself in a way that communicates effectively and creates a fertile practice space for your students. This means knowing when to pull back and moderate yourself. For example:

- If you are the one who always has everyone in the room in stitches, one of your gifts as a teacher is going to be humour. But you may have to be mindful not to fill quiet spaces with jokes, or be funny when a student needs you to be serious. Humour is essential to a fully functioning class container, but you may have to make sure to notice when it might be acting as a shield and actually getting in the way of being real with your students.

- If you are a born researcher with a love of facts and theory, one of your strengths is going to be your capacity to offer information to your students. But you may have to remember that yoga is essentially about individual somatic experience and make sure you don't fill time for experiential practice with words and concepts.

There is room for every kind of teacher, and whichever kind of teacher we are, we need to maintain a degree of balance. If you're not sure whether you're getting this right, a great way to receive feedback is to ask an experienced teacher who you trust to observe you teaching. If you have a long-term relationship with the teacher, they may be able to do this for free, but be prepared to pay. Teaching observation is skilled work, and it's reasonable for the teacher to charge for the service.

EXPERIENTIAL WORK: BREATH

The experiential work for this chapter is short and sweet. This exercise is a simple way to tune in to the pauses that naturally occur within the cycle of your breath. You can do it for 30 seconds when you stop to make a cup of tea, stroke your cat or turn off your computer, or for longer as a formal practice. You don't need any pens, paper or other equipment.

1. Pause and begin to be aware of your breath. Notice the breath coming in...the breath going out... No need to change anything. Just notice your breath as it naturally arises.

2. Now begin to notice that at the end of the in-breath and before the next out-breath there is a small pause...and at the end of the out-breath and before the next in-breath there is also a small pause.

3. Allow yourself to drop into the pauses between in-breath and out-breath, out-breath and in-breath, just resting there momentarily. You don't need to extend the pauses; just let them be as they naturally are.

4. Re-orient yourself to the outside world: notice the sounds around you, what you can see, what you can feel and taste. Notice any changes in your state of being and go on with your day.

The sacred pause

Buddhist teacher Tara Brach offers a simple and powerful daily life practice called 'The sacred pause', which involves creating short pauses in your day. Initially, these might be mostly deliberate and triggered by an alarm; eventually they may become more spontaneous. Tara's 50-minute talk on the value of pausing, in which she also outlines the practice, is recommended listening for anyone interested in cultivating slower living, mindfulness and attention.[11]

4

Ethics, Boundaries and Right Relationship

In this chapter, we will be considering how we can maintain an ethos of integrity in our classes and be the most effective possible container for our students. We will also be looking at some of the ethical issues that may arise in teaching yoga. Central to being an ethical teacher is the ability to create and sustain healthy boundaries between ourselves and our students. When we talk about boundaries, we are essentially considering relationship and how we create it in an appropriate and mutually enlivening way. In the context of student–teacher, the relationship being crafted is a particular and unique one, described by senior yoga teacher Donna Farhi as alchemical in nature:

> In the best possible sense, the teacher acts as a crucible for the student's process of transformation. By necessity, a crucible must be of a harder metal than the element that is being melted. The teacher acts to uphold a safe and sacred container in which the process can occur.[1]

Transference, counter-transference and projection

These three terms originate in psychotherapy. Although they have slightly rarified clinical connotations, they describe some very ordinary ways in which human beings relate to each other, and they will, as a matter of course, be present in the various dynamics that play out between ourselves and our students.

Transference and counter-transference

In a therapeutic setting, transference happens when the client transfers a feeling originally belonging to an early relationship (most often with a mother, father or other parent figure) onto the therapist. Outside the therapeutic context, any person in a role that can be reconfigured as parental may be the recipient of transference, and a teacher is an obvious candidate. You don't have to be emotionally disturbed, mentally ill or the survivor of an abusive childhood to transfer childhood feelings onto adult relationships. We all do this, to a greater or lesser extent, and with varying degrees of awareness. Transference is part of how human beings relate, and when it is met appropriately, it can be a means of resolving and integrating troubling feelings from our deep past.

Counter-transference is the response of the therapist, or other recipient, to the transference. The counter-transference, too, may derive from an early relationship and may be more or less conscious. If your reaction to a particular student feels to you surprising or irrational, or seems to be operating outside your volition, it could be that this is a counter-transference.

As yoga teachers we are not, of course, in the business of making psychotherapeutic assessments; however, it is helpful to be aware that where a relationship is going pear-shaped, transference and counter-transference may be at play. If in relationship to the student you notice yourself feeling like an inadequate nurturer, an over-protective parent, or even an abuser, it may be that you are receiving and responding to a transference. Simply identifying the dynamic and being aware of anything it's triggering in you from your own past will often be enough to enable you to shift on to more honest, realistic and sustaining ground with the student. However, if your own feelings are intense and the counter-transference is complex, you may need to find a professional with therapeutic training to help you unravel, understand and integrate your own responses.

Transference and counter-transference can play out in myriad ways: the challenging student who identifies you with a strict parent (in response to whom you crack down on class boundaries), the flirtatious student who identifies you with a parent who behaved like a lover (in response to whom you start wearing sexier teaching clothes), or the adulatory student who identifies you with an all-knowing parent (in response to whom you pontificate about enlightenment and act like a guru). This is one possible example:

> Tim is a student whose father was negligent and often absent throughout his childhood. He experiences Dwayne, his yoga teacher, as caring and interested

in his well-being, and sometimes confides in him about his past. Dwayne is older than Tim and appears to offer everything Tim never experienced from his father.

Tim has been Dwayne's student for 18 months when he comes off his bike and breaks an arm. He emails Dwayne to explain that he will not be able to come to the class for a few months. Dwayne expresses his sympathy, wishes Tim well, and tells him he will miss him at the class – then gets on with his life. When Dwayne does not get in touch to find out how he's doing, Tim is enraged. He feels betrayed by Dwayne. Eventually he sends Dwayne an angry email, telling him that he is a fraud and that he should be more concerned for the well-being of his students.

Dwayne takes time to reflect on his feelings before responding to the email. He notices a background sense of sadness unrelated to anything actually happening in his life at present. When he attends to it, sadness turns into grief. Dwayne identifies this feeling as originating in his childhood. From as early as he can remember, his mother was ill and depressed and was not able to look after him properly. He often felt that he had been left to fend for himself. He wonders if – unintentionally – he abandoned Tim in a re-enactment of his own childhood past.

As a result of this reflection, Dwayne is able to re-engage with Tim in a clear, straightforward and empathic way, without being drawn into psychological drama.

REFLECTION

■ If you were Dwayne, how would you now respond to Tim? Are there things that Dwayne needs to change? What might be the repercussions in their student–teacher relationship? Be aware that there aren't any right or wrong answers to these questions, just many possible responses.

■ Have you ever transferred feelings from your past onto a teacher? How did they respond? How did the student–teacher relationship develop? Did your feelings about the teacher change over time? What was the outcome for you?

■ Have you ever been aware that a student was transferring feelings from their past onto you? How did you feel about the student? How did you respond? What happened? Are there things you might do differently in a similar situation in the future?

Projection

Just as all human beings transfer and counter-transfer, so we all project. Sometimes our projections are very wide of the mark, and at other times they may hit close to a truth. We may have a total and blind belief in what we are projecting, or we may be more open to the possibility that reality is different from the way we have framed it. While projections arise in settings of all kinds, the yoga class is often a site of intense feelings, and projections formed there can be very potent.

Projection happens when one person affixes to another a belief, attitude or quality that really belongs to the one doing the affixing. Some projections are flattering. It's not unusual, for example, for a student to project guru status onto their teacher, elevating their knowledge, experience and general behaviour onto a plane that the teacher may wish they did actually occupy. Other projections are, to some degree, disturbing:

- Your student secretly hates their body. When you adjust their stance in a posture, they assume this indicates a belief that their body is not good enough, needs to be 'corrected', or is overweight/round-shouldered/too short/too tall, and so on.

- Your student believes that the goal of yoga is to enter into ecstatic states, and they aspire to an out-of-body experience. When you teach about the importance of physical and energetic relationship with the ground, they feel angry and thwarted.

- You believe that yoga is good for everybody and assume that everyone is receiving benefit from your class. When a student tells you their chronic pain is worse after each class and they are switching to Pilates, you feel angry, shocked and disillusioned.

Authenticity is a natural protector against projection. While none of us can entirely avoid being the recipient of others' projections (especially if we regularly stand up in front of groups of people and teach), we can be so fully and honestly ourselves that there are few surfaces for projection to stick to. Where authenticity fails (it will sometimes), an antidote is gentle deflation. For example, if you notice that some students in your class see you as an ally in their quest for bodily perfection, speak about loving and appreciating your body just as it is. Use the language of honouring, accepting and nurturing rather than the language of correcting. Reframe any questions implying that 'improving' the body is a goal of yoga:

Student: How can I get my leg higher in *hasta padangustasana*?

Teacher: It doesn't matter whether your leg is higher or lower. The intention is to be where you are and notice the sensations, emotions and thoughts that arise as you occupy this physical position. Notice what happens if you press through your foot here/rotate your leg this way/extend into your heel/allow this hip to drop/notice your inhale, and so on.

If some of your students have developed an unrealistic idea about how 'enlightened' you are, mark any mistakes you make while teaching. Answer 'I don't know' to questions you can't answer. If it fits your teaching style, use experiences of failing, misunderstanding or falling short as teaching stories. Let your students know that you are human, just like them, only with a slightly longer practice history, and that by practising more, you will all become more fully human, more of the time.[2]

REFLECTION

▦ Are you aware of any projections students have affixed to you? What did it feel like to be the object of this projection? How did you respond? How did your relationship with the student develop? Is there anything you would do differently if you encountered this situation again in the future?

▦ Are you aware of having made projections onto your students? How did you realise you were projecting? How did your attitude and behaviour towards the student change once you had a better sense of the reality of the situation?

▦ Are you aware of having made projections onto your own teachers? What were they? How did the teacher respond? Did you feel their response was helpful? If not, how might they have responded more effectively?

Dual relationship

Yoga teaching boundaries are particularly complex because they potentially encompass a wide range of different relationships. A psychotherapist is always and only ever in a therapeutic relationship with their clients, but this is not the case for a yoga teacher. While some of our students will always be purely and simply our students and we may know little about them personally, others may also be neighbours and members of our local community, colleagues or people we know in some other professional capacity, or pre-existing friends. Then there are those students who over time also become our friends. This means that no single set of boundary guidelines is going to be appropriate for all teachers of all students in all situations. Most of us are going to be called upon to step into different shoes with at least some of our students at different times.

Students who are already friends

I have a tricky situation with a friend attending my yoga class. They are late every week and expect me to come to the door and let them in – and then they make a lot of noise entering the room. They also make jokey comments about me in front of the class. These might be funny in the pub, but they're inappropriate in a yoga class and feel slightly demeaning. I want to offer my friend all the benefits of yoga, but, seriously, this is starting to become a bit much.

Akoya

In some ways this is the most challenging student group to integrate into a yoga class in an appropriately boundaried way – and it is also the group that a beginning teacher or teacher in training is most likely to have in significant numbers among their students.

When a friend comes to a yoga class, we may assume that since we already know them well and have established a relationship of trust with them, we don't need to ask them to fill in all the usual joining forms and sign up to the terms and conditions. Big mistake! Lack of clarity over the agreement that has been entered into has been central to the demise of many a friendship. If you are expecting your friend to pay and to do so by a certain date, this needs to be clear, as do all the other boundaries – around missed classes, booking deadlines, latest class entry times, and so on. If you offer a mate's rate, details of this, too, should be included in your terms and conditions.

Requiring the usual form-filling and agreement process of a friend – and charging them a fee, even if this is a discounted one – is also key to signalling that in this particular context you will be entering into a different kind of relationship. For the duration of the class, and in any interactions around it, you are changing out of your fluffy friendship slippers and into your formal teacher–student shoes. You will be relating to your friend in a different way and will expect them to do likewise with you.

It can be helpful to use the form-filling process to initiate a conversation about boundaries in this new situation. If your friend has no comparable professional experience, the shifts that will be required in your relationship may be something they have not considered – and once they have considered them, they may decide not to join your class. This can be a wise decision and should be respected – even if you 'need' students. Do not underestimate how challenging it can be for a friend to change familiar relationship patterns and see you in a new role – or how challenging it can be to step into and inhabit the teacher role with a friend.

Fiona brought this issue to a mentor group:

> One of my close friends has joined my yoga class. We're used to sitting over a coffee and gossiping together. Now when we go for a coffee, though, he often starts talking about other students in my class. I'm really uncomfortable talking about them in this way. I'm their teacher and it feels all wrong.

Fiona's experience provoked a discussion in the group about the meaning and extent of confidentiality in a yoga class, where students may be risking making themselves vulnerable. (They may fear they will look stupid, will not be fit or flexible enough, will be seen as old or fat, will not be able to keep up with the rest of the class, will get emotional, will be mocked or laughed at by other students, or will be told by the teacher that they are not 'good enough' to take part in the class.) We all agreed that it is neither professional nor respectful to discuss any student with another student – friend or no. Our intention at all times is to honour the willingness of our students to show up on a mat and entrust us with their practice.

Fiona decided that the next time her friend mentioned another student during a private conversation, she would take this as an opportunity for a conversation about confidentiality, professional boundaries and her obligations as a teacher to all the students in her class. She also noticed feeling that she had 'outgrown' gossipy conversations in general, and needed to make a shift away from relating to her friend through criticism and judgement of other people, towards more heart-felt and authentic personal connection.

REFLECTION

■ Have you had existing friends as students? How was it for you? For them? Have any friendships come to grief? How do you feel about this? (Allow your body, not just your mind, to respond.)

How did you go about negotiating terms and conditions with any friends who have come to your class? Did you offer them any special discounts? Did you have any problems with payment and other practical class boundaries?

How has it been to actually teach your friends? Have you felt you can stand in the teacher's shoes with them? Has anything subsequently changed in your relationship as friends?

Students who become friends

It's important to recognise the difference between being friendly towards your students (approachable, relatable) and being friends with your students (you invite them to your birthday party and share intimate details of your life with them). Most of us aspire to the former, but the latter requires judgement and discretion. While it's not necessarily wrong to enter into a friendship with a student, it is wise to pause and consider before making this transition. Some of the questions you may want to ask yourself include:

- How will being a friend of this student affect our student–teacher relationship? Will we be able to continue in student–teacher roles? Do I value this person more as a friend or more as a student? Do I feel deeply drawn into this friendship? Does it *feel* right and appropriate?

- What might the student want, expect or need from being my friend?

- What do I want, expect or need from being friends with this student?

- Does the student understand that there are boundary issues to be considered in the translation from student–teacher to friends? Do they appreciate that if we enter into a friendship, our student–teacher relationship will inevitably shift and change?

- Does the student have me on a pedestal, or are they relating to the real me, with all my human lumps and bumps?

It's important not to under-estimate the power differential that exists between you as the teacher and your students. This is the case even if you yourself feel that you are a very junior teacher, or a down-to-earth and approachable teacher. While this differential may be bigger or smaller between individual students and individual teachers, to some degree it is inalienable and intrinsic to the student–teacher roles. If the student is your peer, the power differential may be minimal (and may also switch over if, for example, in another situation you are their student or client), but if the student is younger than you, new to yoga, low in self-esteem or emotionally vulnerable, the differential can be huge, and these students may have implausible and romantic views of who you are. Some of the unrealistic beliefs students have expressed about me over the years include:

- I get up at 3am every day and practise ashtanga for many hours.

- My physical practice is not affected by my disabilities.

- I have attained a deep spiritual knowledge inaccessible to them.

- I am always kind and generous.

- I have my life totally sorted out.

- I never get angry or upset.

- I never say or do anything ill-judged or unwise.

- I am vegan/eat only raw food/always eat ayurvedically.

Students may also confuse the insights and personal shifts they have experienced in your class with a special potency that you yourself possess, and this may make you very seductive as a friend, with the student desiring to get closer to you so that they can receive more of this very good thing. In this case, it is important to give back to the student their own authority over their practice and over their own self-development.

REFLECTION

- Do you have students who have become your friend? How has this been for you? And for them?

- Have you befriended students and later regretted it? What happened? Do you think they had a realistic view of who you really are as a person (rather than as a teacher)?

- Have any of your students become a close friend? Why do you think this worked? Did you do anything to ensure a smooth transition in the relationship?

Students who are family

Most of the issues that arise in teaching members of your family are the same as those that occur in teaching your friends – only times 10. You may sincerely believe that your dad or your sister would benefit enormously from practising yoga and really want to offer them this gift. However, family roles and dynamics are deeply rooted, and it is prudent to reflect on whether you are the appropriate person to teach your family member. It's also helpful to consider whether you are hoping for a particular outcome from the teaching – your dad will respect your work/your mum will be released from depression/you will develop a closer relationship with your sister/your brother will relax…

Leah brought this dilemma to a mentor group:

> I've started teaching my foster mother one-to-one, and this is bringing up all sorts of unpleasant feelings in me. Since I was fostered, at the age of seven, I've had a difficult relationship with her. I feel as if now the universe is offering me an opportunity to face up to and deal with this relationship, but it's very, very challenging, and I'm feeling quite disturbed. How should I approach teaching my foster mum?

I asked Leah to tell us something about her childhood relationship with her foster mother, and it gradually became evident that it had involved physical and emotional abuse. I invited everyone in the group to offer a response to Leah. Initially, as each person expressed their distress and concern for her welfare, Leah reacted by restating the opportunity she felt the universe was offering her and expressing the belief that it was her responsibility to heal the relationship with her foster mother. Gradually, however, she began to hear what her peers were saying. At the check-out at the end of the meeting, Leah told us she had decided to put a hold on the one-to-one sessions for the time being. Afterwards, she asked about scheduling some Phoenix Rising yoga therapy sessions to explore her feelings about her childhood and perhaps integrate some of the trauma she had experienced.

REFLECTION

- Have you taught members of your family? How did it go? Were you able to be their teacher? Were they able to let go of being your mum/dad/ sister/brother, and so on? Do any body feelings or images come up? Do any old memories get triggered?

■ Are there family members you feel it would be wise not to attempt to teach? What do you imagine might happen?

■ Have you been brought closer to a family member by teaching them? Why did this work? What did you do to enable this expansion in relationship to take place successfully?

Students who are peers

When the student is also a peer, with a similar background, work and life experiences to your own, the transition to friendship can often be easy to negotiate. If you and your student are both experienced yoga teachers, with an understanding of professional boundaries that is not only theoretical but also practical, you may find yourself slipping easily into an unproblematic friendship in which you attend each other's classes, discuss your work and socialise together – perhaps within a broader group of local teachers. I've made lots of friends like this, not only with other yoga teachers and therapists, but also with movement professionals, osteopaths, bodyworkers and the like.

REFLECTION

■ Does your student body include some of your peers? How has teaching peers affected your larger relationship with them?

■ Has teaching peers had an effect on your sense of community? What has changed and how?

Students who are colleagues

The chief complexity in this situation is the possible reversals of rank it may entail, especially if you are actually teaching at work. While some workplaces have a more informal and horizontal culture where status is little marked, others are distinctly vertical. I've taught a workplace class in one organisation for well over a decade now. As a teacher coming in from outside, I'm aware of the manifestations of hierarchy that occasionally play out in the class, but personally I'm outside and immune from them. However, if you have to go back to your desk and work with the boss who felt awkward being a yoga beginner in front of you, or the colleague who boasted all week about how advanced she was at yoga and then fell over in *trikonasana*…there are going to be bumps to negotiate in your professional relationship.

This experience was offered by Anna in an online support group for yoga teachers:

> In one class, I teach my former manager (now retired). Initially, she reverted to manager role and was quite disrespectful towards me. She was rude and even argued with me when I told her not to use the studio mirrors for *viparita karani* for health and safety reasons. She proceeded to state her case by trying to pull the mirror off the wall to prove how stable it was! She would sometimes walk out during final relaxation, making as much noise as possible, which disturbed the other students and made them feel uncomfortable. Before class, she would often complain and would even stand over me as I sat on my mat, telling me what she didn't like.

Anna's response to her student/manager's inappropriate behaviour was to tackle it head on, making it clear to her that in the yoga class setting their former professional power dynamic was not in play and that now, as teacher, she was not prepared to be undermined:

> In the end I asked her to stay after class for a chat. I told her that if she didn't like the class, then she shouldn't attend it. Ever since then she's behaved herself!

Anna's student proved fluid enough to be able to accept the change of shoes – eventually – but it could have gone either way. If your student/superior is really wedded to the status quo, you may have to be prepared to lose them as a student. And if they are your current boss, this may have ramifications for your working relationship.

I have come across a few instances where a newly qualified yoga teacher has ousted the regular yoga teacher offering classes in their workplace, sometimes with the encouragement of colleagues. Please don't do this. Enter your new professional field with respect for those who are already tilling the soil and who may have laboured hard over the years to make it fertile. Yoga teachers often know each other quite well, and this kind of behaviour will certainly be discussed and will play a part in determining your reputation within the local community of teachers. If there is a genuine problem with the existing teacher, this should be discussed with them by the person organising the classes, and where possible, resolved in such a way that the original teacher continues to teach the class.

REFLECTION

- Have you taught your colleagues? How did this go? Was there any rank pulling or awkwardness over the status quo?

- If teaching your colleagues was a success, why do you think this was? What sort of attitudes made the student–teacher relationship possible?

- If teaching your colleagues was not a success, why do you think this was? Did particular attitudes play into the difficulty?

Students within a small community

In London, where I teach, group classes tend to consist of a pretty anonymous group of people. If you teach in a village or small town, on the other hand, it's highly likely that you are already in some kind of relationship with the majority of your students. They may be your doctor, your children's teacher, the assistant in the local shop or your neighbour. In a small community, it's simply not feasible to uphold the kind of professional separation that some city yoga teachers prefer.

A potential flashpoint to look out for if you teach in this situation is breach of confidentiality. When you regularly chat with your students in other contexts, and about all sorts of things, it can be easy to forget that some information may have been shared with you within the protected space of the teacher–student relationship and is not for public consumption. Anwen says:

> I teach in a little rural town, and already knew lots of my students before I started teaching them. I went to school with one of my students – let's call her Linda – who now works as a receptionist at my dentist's. Last time I went for an appointment, we got talking about a mutual friend, also one of my students, who had recently divorced. Let's call him Steve. It wasn't gossip; we were genuinely concerned about him. I started telling Linda about something Steve had told me, and then suddenly remembered that he had mentioned it at the end of a yoga class. It was an insight that had come to him during *savasana*. I realised that it had been told to me in my professional role and that I should have kept it confidential.

REFLECTION

- Do you teach in a small community? What are the challenges?

- What are the gifts, pluses and advantages?

- Have you experienced difficulties with confidentiality?

- Have you been challenged to change to and from different kinds of shoes often and nimbly?

Students with developmental trauma

Students who have experienced significant and unresolved childhood trauma (sustained physical, emotional or sexual abuse and/or neglect) may tend to relate to the teacher as a parent, projecting onto them characteristics that their own parents lacked. As a result, the teacher may become very seductive as a potential friend or lover. To the student you may appear to be the kind, all-nurturing parent, the parent who is always fair, the parent who never abuses them, the parent who is not addicted or depressed, the parent who is available and cares about them, and so on. In fact, most of us project fantasies and beliefs like this onto our teachers, but if we're not traumatised, we generally have greater capacity to recognise our projections as such and refrain from acting upon them. For students with unresolved developmental trauma, the thrust of the parental projections can be very strong indeed, and the capacity to distinguish them from reality quite limited. Careful, kind and determined boundary holding with these students is absolutely essential – and likely to be very challenging.

For more about teaching people with developmental trauma see Chapter 6.

Students with a romantic interest in you

I think one of my students fancies me. He hasn't actually said he does, but he's offered to fix my car and help me with some decorating. I sometimes notice that he's staring at me in class. I find this a bit weird and it freaks me out. He usually stays behind after the class to ask me ridiculous questions – obviously so he can have a chance to talk to me. I'm now giving him the cold shoulder – being curt and saying the minimum necessary when he asks me a question. He hasn't actually done anything threatening. I just don't like his energy much and feel uncomfortable.

Talia

It's very common and absolutely normal to feel sexually and/or romantically attracted to your teacher. As teachers we often represent for our students qualities that they aspire to (sometimes because we do actually embody these qualities and sometimes because the student is projecting them onto us). Students may see us as more realised than they are, more 'spiritual', more disciplined, wiser, more grounded, more centred, more emotionally balanced and, of course, that old favourite, fitter and more flexible. And they may ascribe to us personally any positive transformations they have experienced in our class. All of this is very sexy. Who wouldn't want to get closer to that?

Know that you can expect some of your students to fancy you. It isn't dangerous (unless they are *actually* endangering you in some way – for more on this, see below, 'Sexual harassment by students'), and infatuation can be a healthy stage in the process of embodying the personal changes and recalibrations that come about through practising yoga. Holding people in this phase of development without pathologising or belittling them, and while still maintaining responsible student–teacher boundaries, is an important part of the job of being a yoga teacher. We are duty-bound to support our students in this way and to relate to them with kindness and compassion through the psycho-emotional passages that make up the territory of practising yoga.

In our culture, women are primed to fear certain kinds of sexual/attraction-related behaviour from men. As teachers, however, we need to be established enough in our own two feet – to have sufficient gravitas and adequate outside support – to stand outside the pursuer/pursued trope of male–female relations and go on stably and reliably holding the relational container for the student, irrespective of their gender. This means that we can be with what's happening without being pulled in or getting reactive. We can maintain the necessary boundaries with care not only for ourselves but also for the student.

Being in love with your teacher (or thinking you are) is a vulnerable position. Assuming that the student is not behaving in an aggressive or threatening way towards you (if they are, you need to involve the police), it's best not to shame or discomfort them by confronting them about their feelings and behaviour. Simply hold your boundaries, in the appropriate way. You are their teacher – not their friend, lover or potential partner. You are concerned about their well-being and interested in how their yoga practice is affecting them as a whole person – from the point of view of a teacher.

It can be helpful to name for the student the uniqueness and potency of the teacher–student relationship. While the student may have to lose the dream of a romantic relationship with you, they will be gaining the reality of a deep and sustaining connection, with the potential for deepening and growth.

If you are heterosexual, be aware that your students are quite possibly not, and that in any case teacher crushes can cross the line of expected sexual preference. Don't be blindsided into letting a needed boundary lapse because you had not anticipated that a man/woman/trans/genderqueer person might be romantically attracted to you.

REFLECTION

- What do you do in your own teaching to make sure your boundaries around sexual/romantic relationship are clear and consistent? How has this worked? Have there been misunderstandings? How have you dealt with them?

- Have you ever been sexually attracted to or in love with one of your teachers? How did it feel? Was it just a fantasy or did you hope or believe that you could be in relationship with your teacher in reality?

- Have students been sexually attracted to or in love with you? How did you recognise this? How did you feel about it? Include your body's response now as you remember this experience.

- If the student talked to you about their feelings, how did you respond? Would you respond in the same way again or might you respond differently?

- Has your gender and/or sexuality affected your experiences of love and attraction with teachers and/or with students?

Sexual harassment by students

I've had students invite me on holiday, profess their love for me, ask if I'll be a sperm donor, follow me home, verbally attack me for not becoming their lover, bad-mouth me in the changing room, and tell me what an awful teacher I am and accuse me of not caring because I didn't respond to their advances.

Marcus

It shouldn't go with the territory, but for a yoga teacher this kind of harassment sometimes does – particularly if you work in an environment where a wide range of different people, exhibiting the full spectrum of human behaviour, show up in your class space every day. Senior Iyengar yoga teacher Theresa Elliott cites as one factor in her burn-out after 22 years of teaching yoga, 'handling…the conspicuously aberrant humans and completely unreasonable students who have come my way'.[3] She describes one student whom:

> I had to get an anti-harassment order against. I took her to court and was granted an order of protection, so she retaliated and set up a website defaming me. Last I checked it was still up, and I've used the site for years in my teacher trainings as an example of how yoga teachers are not exempt from unwanted attention and can become targets of harassment like anyone else.[4]

That said, in 16 years of teaching I don't recall ever being sexually harassed, propositioned, sent inappropriate emails or otherwise annoyed by a student. I have had two Phoenix Rising yoga therapy clients fall in love with me, but intense transference is part of the therapeutic process and something we work with in therapeutic relationship. Why is my experience so different from Marcus's and Theresa's? I want to say it's the way I hold the teaching container, but Marcus and Theresa are both very experienced teachers, and it seems unlikely that they don't know how to hold a clear and coherent classroom space. So maybe it's something more personal. I honestly don't know.

If you are being sexually harassed by a student, continue to say no, clearly and evenly. Be polite but blank. If necessary, report the issue to your employer (if you have one). Where a student's unwanted interest is starting to look like stalking, begin to keep records of their interactions with you and involve the police. Stalking is a criminal offence – the Suzy Lamplugh Trust runs the National Stalking Helpline.[5]

REFLECTION

- Have you ever been harassed by a student? How did you feel? How did you respond to the situation? Was it effective? Are there things you might do differently in future?

- Has this experience changed how you hold your class container in any way?

Responding to invitations

There are times when it's absolutely appropriate to accept an invitation from a student. Perhaps you have taught them for a long time and they want to buy you a coffee and discuss teacher training with you. Or perhaps they are a peer and there is a possibility of friendship and collaboration between you. Or perhaps your class is also a community, and it's normal for all of you to head off for a cup of tea together after class. But sometimes an invitation feels in some indefinable way like a date. If you suspect that your student may have sexual/romantic expectations that you cannot meet, don't try to dodge their invitation or fudge things with them. Decline kindly and be clear with the student about why you can't socialise with them. Exemplify honesty and straightforwardness for your student. Don't invent a partner (or harp on about one you do actually have) in order to deter a student who may be attracted to you. Meet their feelings face on and with respect. This is a great opportunity for clarifying boundaries and educating about the breadth and scope of the relationship you do already have with the student as their teacher.

REFLECTION

- Have you ever been offered an invitation by a student? Under what circumstances might you accept an invitation? When would you not?

- Have you ever had to explain to a student the boundaries of the teaching relationship? How did the student respond? Would you do this similarly in future or are there things you would do differently?

Falling in love with a student

I had a relationship with my teacher. It started almost immediately, and I was whisked out of the student role to become a co-teacher – even though at that point I didn't have any teacher training. It was amazing, but I also felt lost. The feelings were very confusing. Even now, separated from my former teacher/partner and trained to teach, I feel that I have missed some important first steps. I'm angry about what my teacher allowed to happen. There's a power dynamic in dating the teacher. It feels so flattering to both parties at the beginning, but it's very difficult to make it work. For me, it all came unstuck.

Ella

The attention of a student who sees you as the kind of wise/enlightened/compassionate/caring/super-fit/unbelievably flexible/knowledgeable teacher that you'd really like to be can be very sexy. Similarly, it can be intensely erotic for the student to be 'chosen' by a person they look up to, regard as perfect, project into a parental role or aspire to resemble. However, such a relationship is built on shaky ground and, as in Ella's experience, can ultimately be very damaging for the student.

While it's inappropriate to date students on a whim or as a serial activity, most of us will know someone who met their life partner while in a teacher–student relationship with them. Maybe this happened to you. Love, like wild flowers, has a way of erupting through unlikely crevices, and it is certainly possible to build a strong sound partnership upon a meeting that first happened as teacher and student – if both parties are firmly grounded in the reality of each other and are aware of the potential distortions created when a power dynamic is in play. If you do experience a deep, genuine and reciprocal connection with a student, it's only sensible to explore it – but make sure you do this within secure professional boundaries. Most teacher registration organisations take the transition from teacher to sexual/emotional partner very seriously and make stipulations about how it should be managed. These often include:

- Sever the student–teacher relationship.

- Take a break from seeing each other. Many professional codes of ethics specify a period of time that should elapse before a former teacher–student duo transitions into a romantic partnership. Check what your registering body requires. This in-between time allows space for cooling off, clarifying feelings and reflection.

- Seek mentoring from a senior teacher.

REFLECTION

- Have you ever been sexually/romantically attracted to a student? How did you boundary and manage this? What worked for you? What might you do differently in future?

When a student discloses sexual abuse by a teacher

If a student discloses to you that another yoga teacher has sexually abused them, the chances are that they feel very vulnerable and don't know who else to turn to. It's important to listen without trying to shut them down. Some sexual abuse may be 'just' unethical: flirting and entering into a casual sexual relationship. Other abuse may be actually illegal: rape or sexual assault.

This situation can be highly sensitive on a number of levels and very tricky to deal with, particularly if, as sometimes happens, the student doesn't want you to say anything to anyone and is not willing to take any action. Sometimes the teacher in question may be a serial offender who is known about in the local community but who has got away with it because victims are unwilling to give evidence to a professional body or to the police.

So what do you do if a student tells you about sexual misconduct by one of your colleagues? I asked a cohort of yoga teachers, and these are the suggestions they came up with.

Unethical sexual behaviour

- Affirm for the student that what the teacher has done is wrong and should not be tolerated, and that they are themselves in no way responsible. Students sometimes become victim to sexual predation because they already have a history of sexual trauma. They may therefore be unclear about what is and isn't acceptable. Even where there is no pre-existing trauma, victims of unethical sexual behaviour commonly experience the shame and guilt that rightly belong to the offender.

- Advise the student to tell the teacher clearly and firmly to stop texting them after the class/touching them in a way they have not invited/ making comments about them during the class, and so on.

- If the sexual behaviour does not stop, advise the student to make a complaint to the gym or studio (if the class is in one of these settings) or to the teacher's professional body (if they have one).

- If the student is very distressed, suggest that they seek help from an appropriate professional trained to work therapeutically with emotional and psychological issues.

Illegal sexual behaviour

- Affirm for the student that the behaviour is wrong.

- Suggest that the student reports the incident to the police. But don't be surprised if they're unwilling and don't pressurise them: it's their choice. Rape victims often describe the process of reporting and going to court as more traumatising than the rape itself.

- Do not attempt to intervene or talk to the offending teacher yourself.

- If the student is not willing to make a report to the police, contact the teacher's employer (if there is one) and/or professional body (if they are registered with one) and tell them what you have been informed about the teacher's behaviour.

- Advise the student to seek help from an appropriate professional trained to work therapeutically with trauma.

REFLECTION

Has a student ever confided in you that they have been abused by another yoga teacher? What did you do? What was the outcome? Is there anything you might do differently if you found yourself in this situation again?

Financial boundaries

I've just set up my first class. I have a box for people to put their class payment in, but on a few occasions, the money has been short. Other times, people have forgotten to bring money and have asked if they can pay next week. I'm not happy about this, but it seems mean to say no.

Alyssa

Establishing and maintaining secure boundaries around money is an important aspect of holding the container of your class, a service you do both for yourself and for your students. As the teacher, you are responsible for ensuring an equal exchange between you and your students, and among your student group. If you don't do this effectively, some students will get away without paying, while others dutifully pay every week, and eventually this will cause bad feeling. Similarly, if you are repeatedly underpaid for your teaching – because someone always 'forgets' to put their money in the box – your positive regard for your students will be undermined. Dealing firmly and fairly in financial matters isn't embarrassing or unpleasant; it's part of being the adult in the situation, the one who takes responsibility and ensures everyone's well-being and safety. It's essential to sitting in the teacher seat.

Good money practices

- Have a system and keep records. This can be an online booking system that you pay for, or it can be a class register in a lever-arch file. Personally, I run my whole teaching business with A4 notebooks and block-booking cards (which I print myself on blank postcards), and payment in cash or by bank transfer. But I do have a system, and I have a record of all the relevant names, dates and payments.

- Ensure that everyone pays in a timely way. Supermarkets don't let you take your groceries home until you've handed over the money. Operate your classes in the same way. Even if your student does pay next week, as promised, the delay entails extra head space and administration on your part – not to mention that for seven days the money is in their bank account, not yours.

- If you offer block-booking options, make the terms and conditions very clear at point of sale, and adhere to them, otherwise your block-booking system will quickly collapse into a free-for-all. I know: it happened to me. Now, no one is saying you need to be a stickler; there is a balance to be struck. Where a student has not been able to use a block-booking for reasons entirely outside their control (serious illness, major injury or family bereavement, for example), most teachers will use their discretion in the student's favour. On the whole, it's best to offer what will encourage the student back into class, such as an extension on the expiry date (rather than a refund). 'Didn't have childcare', 'got my period', 'had to work late', and the like are not valid reasons for a class pass extension.

- If you're offering classes to students who can't afford to pay anything, it's best to require some kind of exchange, even if it's only a token one (decorating, baby sitting, help with setting up before class, book-keeping, for example). Free classes for no alternative investment tend to attract students who neither appreciate nor commit to the class

– and most serious students feel happier about accepting a free class if they can offer something in return. (For more on offering work exchanges, see Chapter 2, 'Setting up your own classes: Pricing'.)

- Unless your class is by voluntary donation, don't have students put their money anonymously into a box or bowl. This sends out the message that it doesn't matter whether people pay and how much, and when there is a non-payment or under-payment (there will be eventually), you won't know who is responsible. This matters because the whole class then falls under suspicion, people start to feel unfairly done by and to suspect each other, and your class dynamic quickly becomes poisonous. Take the money yourself (or have an assistant take it), and make a record of payments. Should you ever have a tax inspection, you will also then be able to demonstrate that you have been diligent in tracking your income.

PRACTICAL WORK: YOGA AND MONEY ETHICS QUIZ

This quiz is intended to be done with a group of yoga teacher friends. Each go through the quiz on your own first, and then compare answers. There aren't any right or wrong ones. The idea is to stimulate discussion, share experiences and get you thinking about different angles on financial matters that might not have occurred to you.

1. Your friend has joined your yoga course. It's three weeks in and they still haven't paid. Do you...

   A. Tell them they're taking liberties and need to give you the money now?

   B. Explain that you are investing your time and energy in the course, that you have costs to cover, and that you need everyone on the course to pay the fee?

   C. Ignore the situation, but continue to feel disgruntled?

   D. Let it go - your friendship is more important, and you're happy to give them something for free?

2. The gym you teach for tells you that it is cutting the fee for yoga teachers to bring it more in line with what they pay fitness instructors. Do you...

   A. Resign immediately. You're worth more than that!?

   B. Take it on the chin. Maybe you were overpaid anyway?

   C. Explain to the gym manager how much training you have done and how much CPD [continuing professional development] you still do, and argue that you are worth the extra money?

   D. Tell all your gym students what has happened and ask whether any of them would be interested in coming to a class you organise yourself?

3. A student who has been coming to your classes for a while loses their job. You don't offer concessions, but they ask if they could pay less for classes for a while. Do you...

   A. Immediately agree. You want yoga to be available to everyone?

   B. Offer them the reduced cost class but request that they help you with setting up and putting away as a work exchange?

   C. Say no – you are concerned about not offering the same deal to other low-income students and wonder if the class would be viable if you gave a special deal to everyone who asked?

   D. Create a concessionary rate that is available for everybody – but don't offer any further reductions on that?

4. Two students who came to a retreat you ran took part in all the classes but clearly didn't have a good time. Now they are asking for half their money back. Do you...

   A. Say no, no way. If they didn't enjoy the retreat, it's their problem?

   B. Worry that they will tell people and create negative publicity, so give them the money back?

   C. Explain that you have a no-refund policy but that you can offer them a 20 per cent reduction on a future retreat?

   D. Have a crisis about your ability as a teacher, worry that no one enjoyed the retreat...and refund the money?

5. A student wants to pay extra for a class. You are getting the feeling that this is because they are sweet on you. Do you...

A. Explain that the class costs X amount and that you don't need anyone to pay any more?

B. Accept the money - they can afford it and you haven't promised anything extra in return?

C. Gently refuse the money and speak about teacher-student boundaries at an appropriate point during the class?

D. Accept the money and ask them out for a drink?

6. A friend tells you that a corporate class they used to teach has come to an end because the organiser wanted them to drop the price. The organiser approaches you and asks if you would take the class on for a lower fee than the original teacher was getting. Do you...

A. Say no - the fee is below the going rate and taking on the class would compromise your relationship with your friend?

B. Say yes - all's fair in love and war?

C. Talk to the original teacher, find out how they feel and decide accordingly?

D. Suspect that the organiser might be a tricky person to work for, sound them out further, also talk to your friend and see what they know, and proceed with caution?

Work phones and email addresses

Good boundary keeping is best served by having a professional phone number and email address (with appropriate signature) and using only these – rather than your personal ones – to communicate with students. This will signal to potential students from the outset what sort of relationship they are entering into with you: that you uphold professional standards, understand and are able to create and sustain healthy boundaries, and can be entrusted with their practice. This kind of professional frontage also acts as a deterrent to people covertly, or not so covertly, soliciting sexual services. Yes, you know the ones.

In my view, it isn't appropriate to communicate with individual students – especially potential new ones – via Messenger, WhatsApp or text message. These are all too informal for the relationship being contracted. If a student messages or texts, direct them to your email address. For example:

Student: I'm interested in your workshop on Saturday. Can I book?

Teacher: Thanks for your enquiry. Yes, you can. Please email joeblogs@ joeblogsyoga.com and I'll send you a booking form.

Separating personal from professional phone and email also means that when you're not at work, you can turn on voicemail and auto-responder and completely switch off. Yes, you can. It's important for your own well-being.

REFLECTION

- How do you communicate with potential new students? Do you have a separate phone number and email address for your teaching work? If so, how has this helped you to maintain appropriate boundaries with your students?

Social media

While in some ways the wonderful world of social media has been a huge enabler in creating teacher visibility and promoting classes, it has also introduced a whole new raft of complexities into teacher–student relationships.

Instagram, Twitter and Facebook

Any of your students can choose to follow you on Instagram or Twitter, even if you feel that you are posting or tweeting on a personal account. This means that you need to be circumspect about any content you put out here. It's totally public. Facebook, on the other hand, involves a mutual agreement to connect. As long as you have your privacy settings tied down, it therefore offers the possibility of a protected social media space which cannot be accessed by your students.

The 'friend' word carries an emotive range of connotations and associations even in the context of Facebook, and it can feel difficult to refuse friend requests from students. In general, however, I feel that it is appropriate to friend students on Facebook *only* if you are using your account solely for professional purposes. If your Facebook account is where you post pictures of your children, chat to your actual friends and express random opinions, it's not a place for connecting with students. Create a page for your work and direct any students who want to friend you there. On Facebook it's possible to adjust your privacy settings so that certain groups of friends see only selected posts; personally I avoid this set-up with students. My feeling is that by accepting a friend request you are giving your student the erroneous message that you are their friend. It's ethical to be clear, transparent and honest on all levels about what the relationship actually is. There are, of course, going to be grey areas: some students verge on real-life friends, and in this case it may be appropriate to 'friend' them, but do this with discretion. The blurring of boundaries that can occur through social media connections with students is real. It can and does affect the way your students see you and relate to you, and can create serious misunderstandings.

A Facebook page is a shop window for your work. Facebook groups can also be a good way to communicate with particular sections of your student body and can enable students to communicate with each other. I have a group for my Mysore practitioners, a group for people who dance with me at Greenwich Moves, a group for people who dance with me in the urban wild, and so on.

WhatsApp groups

Teachers are increasingly using WhatsApp groups to engage informally with their students – to remind them of upcoming workshops, share photos and videos, and this kind of thing. It should go without saying, but perhaps doesn't, that you should not be participating in a professional WhatsApp group with your students on a personal phone number.

REFLECTION

- Which forms of media (if any) are you currently using to communicate with your students? Are they serving your needs? Are they serving your students' needs? Are there any issues with boundaries? Or with confidentiality?

- Have you experienced any difficulties or misunderstandings that could perhaps have been avoided if you had used different media to communicate?

- Are there forms of communication that are working well for you? Why is this?

Classes or communities: what are you holding as a teacher?

Different teachers have different orientations to their student body. While some maintain a strictly teaching relationship with their students, others are interested in creating and sustaining community beyond the yoga mat.

When I first began teaching I related to all my students purely, and pretty heterogeneously, as their teacher. If you're a new teacher and have limited experience of negotiating complex professional boundaries, it's not a bad idea to err in this way on the side of safe and conservative. Over the years, however, as I've got older and more experienced at holding people in many different practice settings, this has changed. While forms and structures for working with the body in movement remain for me an essential catalyst and container, I've also become engaged with fostering community that extends beyond practice.

In this role, the teacher functions as the guy rope that anchors and enables a complex webbing of threads between themselves, their colleagues, their assistant teachers and apprentices, and various practitioners in various different teaching and practice settings. We all know each other in many different ways, and this creates a kind of relational composting, bringing richness to all our soil.

Being this kind of teacher requires a capacity for relational fluidity together with discretion and discernment. It's less like a rule book and more like an improvised dance in which the steps may be strange and surprising but on a felt level are just 'right'. You are still held within the container of ethical relationship. You still don't have casual sex with your students. You still determine who it's appropriate to enter into intimate friendship with and who it really isn't. You still maintain confidentiality. Being in community with your students doesn't mean that you are no longer upholding appropriate professional boundaries.

Neither of these approaches towards relating to students is better than the other, but one or the other may be more appropriate in particular situations, places, times or phases in a teaching life. You may find you have a natural leaning towards one approach over the other: some teachers are natural and consummate communitisers, whereas others prefer to stick only to teaching and not complexify their relationship with their students further.

For more on building community see Chapter 8, 'Creating practice communities'.

REFLECTION

▣ Are you a communitiser? What would be your idea of a well-functioning, sustaining practice community – even if you are not in a position to enable one now?

▣ Do you uphold relatively strict boundaries with students? What are your reasons for choosing this way of relating to them?

▣ Whether you are a communitiser or a teacher-only, can you envisage situations where your orientation might shift? Why might this be? How might it feel to shift your role in this way?

Holding a balanced container

I teach in a small gym where most of the students have never done yoga before. The gym encourages me to offer students the kind of class they want, so I always ask them what they would like. Last week, they said they wanted a fast, sweaty class, so I did dynamic vinyasa, but at the end they were dissatisfied and said they wanted to stretch more. Next time, I did a class with some yin postures in it, but that didn't seem to be what they wanted either. I'm getting really confused. What do my students actually want?

Aarti

Aarti's experience demonstrates what can happen when the teacher does not stand in their own feet and the job of holding the container is passed over to the students. An effective teacher creates a space in which there is permission and there are also clear and tangible boundaries. When people come to a yoga class they may express all sorts of desires, wishes and aspirations, but what they really need on a fundamental level is this kind of holding.

There's a creative tension that holds a good class container in being. On the one hand, an effective class has a sense of cohesion – of the group moving on a similar trajectory and with a similar purpose. On the other hand, at the heart of any yoga class is the invitation to pay attention to somatic experience and proceed on the basis of the information it offers (listen to your body). When there is insufficient cohesion, the group feels disparate and random; people may start following their own choreography, arrive and leave at odd times or chat during the practice. When too much emphasis is placed on unity of trajectory and purpose, the class can feel like a military two-step. In this class, everyone has to do things in the same way. The teacher may have rigid rules about alignment and expect everyone to follow them.

Like a skyscraper, a balanced class has a strong frame but is made of flexible material. It is constructed to sway with the wind without falling apart. If students push they can feel that they are securely held within the class boundaries. At the same time, the teacher welcomes individual somatic expressions of all kinds and is able to weave these into a coherent whole. There is space for students to honour their own needs while at the same time feeling that they are part of the joint enterprise of the class.

Valuing the rebels

Jo was a really difficult person who came across as aggressive and seemed to be challenging me all the time. There was just something about the way they looked at me, and they always seemed reluctant to do anything I asked. I often arrived to teach hoping they would not be in the class. One day, I gave Jo some verbal feedback and they just stormed out of the class. When I got home, they had sent me an email. It turned out that Jo was gender-fluid, and I had been misgendering them. I apologised by email, but Jo never came back to my class. However, I have learnt some valuable lessons. I no longer make assumptions about a person's gender. And if someone is reacting badly to my teaching, I'm much more likely to question what I'm doing and talk to them about it, rather than assuming that they're just difficult.

John

I've often been indentified as rebellious or anarchic. The truth is, I'm autistic. I don't process information in the same way as allistic (non-autistic) people, and I don't see things in the same way either. I have no particular intention to upset the apple cart, but where neuro-normativity is tacitly in place, I will lob a few apples around to make myself some breathing space. Rebellious students may invoke feelings of anger, self-doubt and the desire to 'crack down' in their teachers. However, the rebel is an important person in your class. Often, like Jo, they are holding out for something you have excluded or unwittingly pathologised.

Rebels can expand our ideas. They may be pushing the edges to see whether the container is strong enough to hold them. Often they deeply desire to be included in a way that is neither wounding nor compromising of their integrity. In a truly inclusive and respectful space, the rebel dissolves because there is nothing to rebel against. A skilful and experienced teacher simply goes on holding whatever arises without reacting against it. Not much knocks them off kilter, and students' projections just don't land. In this kind of class container, everyone can relax and all parts of all of us can come to the party.

The informal student contract

Yesterday was lovely weather, so I spontaneously decided to take my class outside. Unfortunately, three of my regular students weren't happy about this. I suggested that if anyone didn't want to go out, we would all stay indoors, but two of the three students decided to leave. It felt really tricky. I'm afraid I have upset people who have supported my class. Should I have handled this differently?

Jilly

When you change a fundamental aspect of a regular class, you are altering the informal contract you have with your students. Rather than presenting everyone with a *fait accompli*, contact your group in advance to let them know what you are planning. Giving everyone an opportunity to opt in or out shows respect for the needs of your students and is important for the energetic holding of the class. A student confronted with an activity they are not comfortable with may not want to be a wet blanket, and rather than spoiling everyone else's fun may leave (or stay reluctantly) feeling alienated. By the same token, there may be occasional students on your list who would have loved to attend the special event if only they'd known about it.

Situations that may warrant advance notice include:

- Taking an indoor class outside or an outdoor class inside.

- Introducing partner work into a class that does not usually involve it.

- Making a dynamic class slow, gentle or restorative – or making a slow, gentle or restorative class dynamic.

- Teaching a completely different style of yoga from the one usually practised.

- Introducing a lot of self-practice into a taught class – or leading a self-practice class.

- Including children in a class that is not usually family-friendly.

Bear in mind that people may have allergies to seeds and pollen in the summer outdoors; they may not feel safe being touched by strangers; they may want quiet space away from children in a yoga class; they may want to work out – or to rest – in their practice; they may hate Dharma Yoga… So be transparent, well in advance, and avoid upset, disgruntlement and diplomatic incidents.

Ethical policies

While most yoga teachers honestly intend to behave ethically, we all have blind spots, and most of us are capable of fudging an ethical matter where it seems harmless and something (or someone) we deeply desire is involved. This is where being signed up to an external system of accountability is invaluable. If you're a member of a professional association, the chances are that you are already bound by a code of conduct. Make sure you've read it and understand what you have committed to. Most ethical codes cover right relationship with students (and colleagues), fair and transparent financial dealings, giving access to classes without discrimination, and scope of practice.

One seminal ethical policy is the 1995 Code of Conduct written by the California Yoga Teachers Association (CYTA) (headed up by Judith Lasater) and published in *Yoga Journal*. The CYTA Code was a response to ongoing misbehaviour by a significant number of yoga teachers occupying elevated positions – a situation that is depressingly still familiar more than 20 years on. Clearly, codes of conduct have leverage only on those who consider themselves bound by them, which super-star and guru-style teachers mostly do not. Judith Lasater writes in *Yoga Journal*:

> Many of the classical teachings of yoga translated well into our culture, but some did not. One area in which there was sometimes an unfortunate gap was in the way the ethical teachings of traditional yoga were understood and practised by Westerners and sometimes abandoned by Indian teachers when they taught in the US… Those of us who are acquainted with the various systems of yoga know of cases of serious ethical violations at some level in

all of the systems of yoga currently taught in the US today. These ethical violations include, but are not limited to, serious cases of emotional, physical, sexual, or verbal abuse.

If you are in search of an ethical lodestone, the CYTA Code of Conduct still covers all the bases and is well worth consideration.[6]

Internal ethical locus

While codes of ethics are central to our integrity as teachers, equally so is what Donna Farhi refers to as our 'internal locus' for ethical behaviour.[7] This is our capacity to intuit in an ongoing way what is ethical with particular students, at particular times and in particular situations. An internally located ethical sense is particularly important in the realm of what Kylea Taylor calls 'nonordinary states of consciousness'.[8] These include states that yoga teachers routinely work with, such as 'deep relaxation and peace' and 'meditation and deep concentration', as well as others that may arise less frequently but will certainly be present at some times in our classes, for example, 'unitive or cosmic consciousness', 'emotionally charged imagery', 'intense energy release' and 'trauma re-enactment'.

The majority of everyday ethical decisions we are called on to make in our classes are not clear-cut but are judgement calls, in which our reading of the situation and our life experiences are required to inform us about what is going to be the most helpful and supportive way to be with the student. A friend of mine is a Feldenkrais teacher. One of her clients is 92. She has been working with him in his home for over 15 years and describes him as 'an old-fashioned gentleman'. Every Valentine's Day he gives her flowers – which she gracefully accepts. On the other hand, Scott, a yoga teacher in mentoring, says:

> I have a student who I know fancies me. I just get that vibe. He recently returned from holiday and brought me a bottle of wine. If it had been a different student, I probably would have said 'thank you' and accepted the present as a mark of appreciation, but with this student I had the feeling there was more at stake. I thanked him for thinking of me and explained that as his teacher I couldn't accept a gift. I told him how much I valued him as a student and explained that I didn't want to jeopardise that relationship in any way.

REFLECTION

▓ Are you signed up to a professional code of ethics? If so, are you familiar with what it contains? Has having this external ethical foundation served you in any way? If you are not signed up to a code of ethics, are there reasons for this?

▓ Has your internal locus for ethics ever overridden an ethical behaviour stipulated in your ethical code? What happened? In hindsight, do you still feel that you did the ethical thing?

The ethics of touch

Touch is one of the foundations of my own teaching practice. I'm deeply engaged by the relational possibilities that arise for teacher and student when touch is included as a possibility in our shared work. As human beings we are essentially tactile and without touch we cannot thrive. At the same time, touch is highly regulated in our culture, and largely hived off and apportioned solely to sex, often in a commodified and domination-oriented form. Many people are therefore hungry for touch that is nurturing, companionable, sustaining and friendly.

As a culture we are in a phase of awakening to the prevalence of abusive touch and to the ways in which touch in the yoga room can refer to and trigger memories of physical and sexual trauma – or can actually be abusive in itself. Central to being an ethical teacher is an awareness of the possible meanings of touch and of our responsibility to touch with respect, wisely and well. There is a potential shadow side of this awareness, however; in some yoga environments, it can feel as if touch itself has become suspect, mindfulness of how we speak through our skin has been replaced by fear and aversion, and touch has been outlawed from teaching practice.

Touch is a complex, multivalent language. Being a tactile teacher does not mean that I am always touching everybody all the time, but that in my understanding we are all always navigating relationships where there is a potential for tactility, and that if our yoga practice is a laboratory in which we research the whole of our life, questions of touch are going to arise here. In a yoga class, this could present as a student choosing to decline touch. A significant part of my work consists of exploring with students and clients the possibility that they have control over when and how they are touched and that they have absolute permission to refuse or modify the physical contact that is being offered – without fear of offending or displeasing.

Different teachers work in different ways and have different orientations to the use of touch as a teaching tool. It's fine to work predominantly verbally or through demonstration if this is a choice that arises from a position of comfort with negotiating and including touch rather than from fear and disempowerment in this area. If you feel that you are lacking this confidence, it would be wise, in my view, to explore touch in your own practice, with your own teachers, and perhaps therapeutically, too, before entering a body-centred profession.

Creating a collaborative culture

Consent to touch is not simple and one-time but is a process – an ongoing communication. It also cannot always be taken at face value. Both in my therapeutic work and in the Mysore room, I am often aware that a client or student is not in a position to give meaningful consent, perhaps because they are in awe of the teacher/therapist and want to please them, or because they believe the teacher/therapist knows best what is good for them, or because they have experienced childhood sexual abuse in which survival depended upon allowing another person complete and unrestricted access to their body. In this situation, any work with touch centres upon repeated communication that the client/student is in charge of what happens to their body. Over-compliance in hands-on teaching is generally a signal to back off – genuine consent has not been achieved – and perhaps, if the student is interested in deeper work with touch and consent, to refer to a body-based therapist, somatic therapist, Phoenix Rising yoga therapist or the like with training in developmental trauma work.

Even where there is no personal trauma, many historical and cultural factors contribute to our expectations of teacher–student relationships in the yoga class and of how permission operates around touch. These include the guru tradition as understood and interpreted by Western people, and our experience of teachers in our own education. On the whole, our norm is an authoritarian set-up, in which the teacher knows the 'correct' answers and tells everyone what to do. As an ashtanga teacher, working within a guru-based tradition, one of the ways in which I attempt to reframe and horizontalise the structure before the student even walks through the Mysore room door is by having a mission statement on my website. It goes like this:

My interest is in working with people within the laboratory of practice. My orientation is somatic, which means that I welcome in everything we encounter through the medium of the body: thoughts, emotions, memories and the dimension of being that is bigger than our own single self. I invite you to listen to your body, honour your experience and understand what happens on your mat in the context of your whole life.

In ashtanga vinyasa, the set form – the sequence of postures – is the bones of the practice. It acts as a container: a crucible within which we can experiment and explore, and the alchemy of yoga can take place. At the same time, we each arrive on our yoga mat with a unique body, a unique background and unique life circumstances, so there must be some flexibility in how we meet with the form so that each of us can enter by a door that makes the practice accessible to us on any given day.

My intention as a teacher is to be in a dialogue with you, sometimes through words, sometimes through touch or breath or energy. I want your feedback; I want to know what's happening for you. I may encourage you if you are scared, but I will never coerce you to do anything, and you are invited to let me know at any time if you don't want to be adjusted, or if an adjustment is too strong or just not working for you. I want your practice to empower you, and I hope that we can be in creative partnership.

As well as signalling to students that they are a partner in a joint enterprise, the mission statement also helps to remind me of what I'm in the room for and what the teaching of yoga is really all about.

Ask before you adjust?

Most often the ways we seek and give consent in relation to the body are not verbal. While asking in words is frequently a part of gaining meaningful consent, it's not the whole story. Just because you've asked and they've said yes, it doesn't mean you have real consent; and you may have requested and received full consent without uttering a word.

Sometimes I ask verbally before I adjust and sometimes I don't. A myriad of factors play into this choice: how well I feel I'm reading the person's needs in the moment, how well I know them, where we are in our practice process with this particular posture, what I'm feeling on a somatic level as I enter their space, whether they have a history of trauma, whether they have a history of injury, whether they are hypermobile, whether they sometimes do/sometimes don't want physical assists, and so on. Similarly, I often ask how the person is experiencing the adjustment – but not always. Sometimes asking in words yields important information, and sometimes it feels as if words get in the way.

More important to me than individual one-off permissions is that I am always seeking to create a culture of choice and exploration in which teacher and student are in partnership. For me, the chief intention of a yoga teacher is the cultivation of relationship. The postures are a structure for enabling this relationship in an embodied way. They are important, but they are not the yoga, and teaching them is not what I am ultimately there for.

Permission cards

Permission cards can have a role in signalling that in your class primacy is given to the student's preferences about touch. They can also be helpful for students who know that they may be unable to refuse consent if asked verbally. This is especially the case if you are in a teaching situation where it is not possible to explore consent slowly and sensitively with individual students.

That said, personally, I don't use permission cards, and the possibility of being offered one as a student fills me with panic. Partly this is because I need the subtle negotiation that happens around physical touch. For me, there isn't a simple yes/no answer; it depends on who and when and how, and I can't predict any of that until it happens. I fear that my body would be fixed by the card into a decision made ahead of time by my cognitive mind, which doesn't – or shouldn't – actually have authority in this area.

Theodora Wildcroft's 'Trauma sensitive' is a good article on consent/permission cards.[9]

For more on touch see Chapter 3, 'Touch'.

Appropriate clothes

My teacher always said that the clothes we wear to teach should give a professional impression. However, that doesn't mean they have to be boring, or that you can't wear bright colours or express your personality and style. Clothes should be clean, not see-through, and without slogans or images that might offend someone or be distracting. What you wear should draw attention only to what you are teaching.

Frankie

As yoga teachers we are working closely with other people's bodies and (potentially) using touch, so we need to take care to dress in a way that signals appropriate professional boundaries. Imagine how you would feel if your doctor showed you into the consultation room in a mini-skirt and a leopard-skin bikini top. We expect to be assured through the demeanour and dress of our doctor that their interaction with our body is not sexual – or maternal or coloured by any emotional responsivity other than empathy and compassion. The same goes for all professionals who work with the body. This doesn't mean that you can't express your individual style and personality through the colours, shapes and combinations of garments you wear, or that you shouldn't choose clothes that allow you to move freely and keep your body temperature regulated; it does mean that you should avoid anything overly skimpy, revealing, salacious or overtly sexualised. This will send a clear signal to your students about the kind of relationship you are engaging in with them, and will help to avert approaches from those who want something different. What you choose to wear sends important signals to your students about your professionalism.

Scope of practice

It seems pretty obvious, but a yoga teacher is trained to teach yoga. Yoga class? What it says on the tin: learning the practice of yoga. 'Yoga' is a vast discipline including many spheres of knowledge and practice. Teaching it requires an equally broad base of skills and range of capacities. If you have completed a 200- or 500-hour teaching certification, you're probably aware of the constraints on what you can learn in this very short time. 'There's so much I still don't know' is the mantra of choice for many newly qualified teachers. However, our students are mostly not aware of this and often believe that yoga teacher training is far more lengthy, thorough, extensive and rigorous than it actually is. If you haven't yet met a student who thinks you know more about medicine than their doctor, or more about biomechanics than a physiotherapist, don't worry, they're coming soon!

Perhaps some of our students' confusion arises from the enormous range and diversity of expertise among yoga teachers. An elder teacher with decades of experience and trainings in several related areas may have a wealth of specialist therapeutic knowledge and a capacity to work in depth with movement patterns, and may indeed be able to spot what a doctor or othopaedist hasn't noticed. However, the demographic of yoga teachers at present is such that the vast majority of teachers do not fall into this category.

Refer, refer, refer

One of my off-and-on ashtanga students contacted me the other day in a bit of a panic. She had discovered what she thought was an umbilical hernia. She wanted me to do an assessment and help her to modify her practice to work with this. I told her that she needed to see her doctor. I do know how to rehab a hernia, but not without medical clearance. An umbilical hernia needs proper diagnosis and usually surgery. It wouldn't be ethical for me to work with a student without this. A lot of damage could be caused, and it could even be dangerous.

Gaynor

New teachers in particular sometimes tell me that they feel they are failing their students if they refer them to other more experienced or specialist teachers. You are not. It is professional to explain honestly to students that you do not have the knowledge or experience to work with them but can suggest someone else who does. Likewise, while we as yoga teachers may often strongly suspect, based on our experience and knowledge, that a student's difficulties derive from a particular condition or dysfunction, we don't have the professional tools to ascertain that this is so. These belong to doctors, physiotherapists, osteopaths and the like. Appropriate referral to a diagnosing professional will expand what we can safely offer the student in terms of their yoga practice and enable us to work with them much more effectively.

I refer often and extensively. I maintain a list of local movement and therapeutic professionals and specialist yoga teachers who I know and trust and can refer to with confidence. What goes around comes around. If a professional I refer to feels that one of their clients would benefit from yoga, yoga therapy or movement work, they may well also refer them to me.

If you are a new 200-hour teacher, you are qualified to work with people who are not currently injured or suffering from complex health conditions, and who have no special needs. Students who are pregnant, have cancer, are elderly and debilitated, are under 14, are traumatised, are mentally ill, have other than very mild back/knee/hip conditions (this list is not exhaustive)…all need to be referred to a specialist or experienced teacher. As a rule of thumb, if, as a new teacher, you feel you need to ask advice before teaching a student, you probably should refer them. You will have enough to think about meeting the normal needs of average students in your class. A more experienced teacher when presented with a health condition they are not familiar with will probably have the capacity to research, seek mentoring, discuss with the student (and perhaps do a simple assessment), and incorporate them into the class, depending on the nature of what needs to be included and the style and size of the group.

It's not only medical conditions and injuries that may require referral. Energetic experiences can require specialist input too. Jake brought this experience to a yoga teacher mentor group:

> I think one of my students is having a *kundalini* awakening. He said at first he felt as if he had been suddenly lifted off the floor. Strange feelings in his body have continued. Sometimes he is elated and at other times he is terrified, and generally he is all over the place. He says he is making some very bad decisions. This is all foreign to me, and I don't know how to advise him.

Jake's peers felt that this student needed guidance from a teacher who had had similar experiences and integrated them. It can be hard to locate such teachers: one of the hallmarks of a genuine awakening is reluctance to draw attention to it. Fortunately, one member of the group knew a teacher who worked with *kundalini* experiences and was willing to meet with the student. Three months later, Jake told us:

> The student seems much calmer and more settled. He told me it was really helpful to talk to someone who had had similar experiences and survived! The teacher told him that *kundalini* is a natural part of all of us, but most of us never encounter it. If you do, there's nothing to worry about. You haven't gone mad. Everything is okay. In fact, you are very privileged. He is continuing to work one-to-one with the teacher. I'm really relieved. I was out of my depth and couldn't offer the student the right kind of support.

Other modalities in the yoga class

Many yoga teachers are also experienced practitioners of other forms of work – aromatherapy, Traditional Chinese Medicine, reflexology, yoga therapy, psychotherapy, massage, and so on. Be aware that people in a yoga class have given consent for you to teach them yoga – only that. If you feel that your other work might benefit a student, talk to them about it after the class, and if they're interested, make a separate appointment. The yoga class is not an appropriate container for other kinds of work, and the student has not agreed to receive it, even a little bit.

REFLECTION

- Do you refer students? Who might you refer and why? Have you ever not referred a student and regretted it?

- If you do other forms of work, how do you handle referring students to yourself? Do you set boundaries around how and when you do this?

- Have you ever felt out of your depth with a student? What happened? Did you resolve the situation? How? If not, what happened? How might you handle a similar situation in the future?

Setting boundaries around student time

I have a student who keeps me talking forever at the end of every class. The class finishes at 10pm, and by that time, I just want to go home and go to bed, but he just doesn't seem to get the message, and I don't feel that I can interrupt him.

Sherrell

As teachers, we want to be available to our students for questions and sharing of experiences related to their practice. I end most classes by saying: 'If there's anything you want to ask or tell me, please feel free to come and talk.' However, we also need to set reasonable limits around how much of this kind of time we offer to our students, otherwise we risk becoming depleted. Being in service to our students does not mean giving ourselves away to them, but modelling clear, fair boundaries that allow space for them but also protect our own needs. If you are exhausted after a class and need to get some sleep, make this clear to anyone who wants to talk at length:

It's been a long day, and I'm very tired. I need to bring this conversation to a close now and go home. See you next week.

Then move towards the door and don't respond to any more conversational gambits. Be honest. Don't say, 'It's been lovely to chat' if it hasn't, because this will suggest to your student that their meandering after-class conversations are welcome.

Notice when offering a few simple pointers after a class is turning into a one-to-one session. This often happens when a person has an injury or condition and needs particular modifications. Value your time appropriately.

If what's required is more than you can offer in five minutes, suggest some individual paid-for time. Say something like:

> This injury is having quite a big impact on your practice. There isn't really time after class for us to go through all the modifcations you need to know to make the group class safe and beneficial. Would it be possible for you to book a one-to-one session?

Or:

> These are great questions. We would need to work together in detail in order to unpick them. If you'd like to book a one-to-one appointment to do that, let me know and we can arrange a time.

For more on this, see Chapter 8, 'Dealing with requests for free advice'.

EXPERIENTIAL WORK: TOWARDS AND AWAY

In this exploration we will be looking at the subtle impulses to move towards... or away from different people. These impulses are rooted in our animal body and form the basis of our inter-personal boundaries. They happen instantaneously and often outside our conscious awareness - before any evaluation based on personality has had time to kick in.

You will need:

- ◉ Thirty minutes of time in a public space where there are plenty of people moving around (art gallery, shopping centre, jumble sale, etc.).

1. Wander around your chosen space for a while and get comfortable with the environment.

2. Now, when different individuals approach, start to notice how you feel as they come closer. Notice your physical sensations: the hairs on the back of your neck, the feeling in your gut. How do you feel as they move away? How do you feel when you are the one moving? Is this different? If it's appropriate to the setting, choose a person (for example, someone in a group around a painting) and deliberately move closer to them. Notice where your comfortable edge is.

3. When you're done, take some quiet time to sift through your experiences. What did you notice? What was familiar to you? Did anything surprise you? Could you predict who you felt drawn towards/repelled away from? What did you learn?

Doing this work as a group

If you belong to a yoga teacher mentor group or meet-up and you have a room with a bit of space, you can do this exploration together.

1. Choose a facilitator (this role can rotate).

2. Everyone walks around the room. Take a minute or so to do this.

3. When the facilitator says 'approach', everyone moves towards another person and stops about a metre away from them. Notice what you feel. Do you want to move closer or move away? Are you aware of any physical sensations? Don't say anything to the other person or communicate to them what you're feeling. Just stay neutral. If there's an odd number and you are left alone, notice the sensations and feelings that go with this. The facilitator gives about a minute for this stage.

4. When the facilitator says 'change position', both partners begin to adjust to a comfortable distance between each other. Let this be a moving exploration as each person moves in and out. Sometimes a tiny shift can make a huge difference. Sometimes you may want to move very, very close; sometimes the other end of the room may not be far enough. There will be partnerships in which each person has a very different sense of how close they want to be. Notice how you negotiate this with your body. Do you give in and go with the distance the other person wants? Do you keep trying to find a compromise? Do you lose all sense of your own body boundary? This is an exploration, so anything can happen. Nothing is right or wrong.

5. When the facilitator says 'pause', everyone bows to their partner (this is important - don't leave it out) and starts to circulate again. At this point, if necessary, the facilitator can jump in and someone else can jump out to take their place.

6. Repeat this process a few times.

7. Come together in a sitting circle and take some time to share your experiences. Each person has an opportunity to speak, if they want to. Keep it anonymous; don't identify any of your responses with particular people. Speak in the first person, about your own experiences only. The rest of the group just listens and witnesses. This is not a conversation.

8. When everyone who wants to has spoken, allow listening and witnessing to shift to a general discussion of towards and away, physical boundaries, and how they play into your role as a yoga teacher.

5

Keeping It Safe

CREATING GENERATIVE SPACES

In this chapter, we will be exploring safe-enough teaching practice. We will be asking what it actually means to feel and be 'safe' in a yoga class, and will also be considering where the desire to keep people safe may impinge on their need for a degree of risk. We will also be considering our scope of practice, looking at working safely with people with health conditions, and considering injury in yoga classes. Holding good boundaries and teaching in an ethical way are, of course, fundamental to safe teaching practice, and this chapter should be read in tandem with Chapter 4.

Safe enough

On an animal level, we are conditioned in a deep and thorough-going way by how safe (or not) we feel in relation to our environment and to the people in it. When we feel safe enough – when threat to our life or well-being is minimal and infrequent – we are able to communicate freely; to input our thoughts, feelings and ideas; to learn, to create, to trust and to take measured risks. In general, there is potential for self-expansion. Conversely, where threat is ongoing and omnipresent, we may retract, hide, retreat, dissemble and withdraw in order to protect ourselves. We may become hypervigilant. Our body may contract and our muscles may brace, sometimes to the point where it's hard to breathe.

Sufficient safety is a prerequisite for a generative teaching space in which students are willing and able to explore. This may sound obvious, but the history of yoga throws up many instances where teaching spaces and teacher–student relationships have been not only unsafe but also outright abusive.[1]

If you're reading this book, it's highly likely that your sincere intention is to create supportive, safe-enough practice opportunities for your students, but we're all flying with a selective radar. This chapter may suggest some ways in which you can feed the soil of your teaching ground so that it is nourishing for every student's learning and exploration.

Safety in the tissues

Having sufficient safety is important not just on a personal level but also on a biological one. My colleague, ashtanga vinyasa teacher Andy Gill, says:

> When the body feels safe and stable, the soft tissues can relax and surrender, allowing the body to become more flexible without straining, and the practice to take on a relaxed and effortless quality.[2]

While we want to encourage our students to try things and expand the edges of what they can do, we also need to take care that there are always solid foundations in place. This is especially important where students are more flexible than strong – bear in mind that in many yoga classes there is a high proportion of hypermobile students. It's important not to press for lots of extensibility without good support. When the tissues are overly challenged, the result may be chronic pain or acute damage, with muscles going into spasm in an attempt to protect and stabilise – not the situation we are aiming for![3]

Expanding our students' capacity

If you've been teaching for a while, you have probably taught at least one person whose response to pretty much any sensation in their body is fear and retreat. My student Julia was like this. When she had a twinge in her back, she completely stopped both folding forwards and bending backwards. And twisting. The focus of her practice seemed to be on propping herself thoroughly enough to avoid any movement at all. While it's generally a good idea to practise away from injury and towards healing the physical body, for Julia, caution and apprehension had taken over to such an extent that they were in themselves becoming harmful, and the range of her movement was growing ever smaller.

When a person is very fearful, it's a priority to develop a relationship of trust. Without this, any suggestions about how they might modify their approach are likely to be rejected. Julia was fairly new to my class, so at first, I mostly just observed her practice, listened to what she said about her back, helped her to feel physically supported by bolsters and blankets, and got to know her better. In this way, I learnt that (like many people) Julia had a belief that any part of her body that was experiencing discomfort needed to be completely rested – that is, immobilised – in order to recover from the 'injury'.

If a student is experiencing serious or persistent pain, it is, of course, important to refer them to a professional, such as a physiotherapist, who can do a proper assessment. Most often, though, what our students report are routine aches and pains which are the result of over- or under-use, or of over-reliance on a particular biomechanical pattern or set of patterns at the expense of physical fluidity. These situations actually *need* intelligent movement in order to resolve. Even where an injury has been diagnosed, standard advice these days generally includes keeping the affected body parts in appropriate motion. For Julia it was helpful to have the therapeutic possibilities of movement named, and her discomfort reframed as useful information, normal and workable in a yoga practice, and part of the process of somatic investigation we are engaged in in a yoga class. It was also helpful to articulate caution–risk as a continuum available for exploration, one presenting a spectrum of possible choices. At some times it might feel appropriate to choose the least possible risk, and at others to be more experimental, the aim being to develop awareness of what we are choosing, and flexibility in the range of choices we are able to make.

Safe enough to take a risk

A key skill of a yoga teacher is being the safety that enables a nervous student to take a reasonable, calculated risk. While we don't force anyone to do anything they don't want to, we do support people as they shed old, tight skins. Bebe was a fairly experienced ashtanga practitioner who really wanted to be able to stand on her head but was also terrified. For many months, I worked on headstand incrementally with her, at first offering a lot of physical and emotional support and gradually withdrawing so that she was increasingly self-sustaining in the posture. A large part of my work involved holding the traumatic feelings of fear that initially emerged as Bebe approached *sirsasana*. I did this just by receiving them kindly, without drama and without attempting to interpret them or make them go away. It was important to keep bringing Bebe back to a safe place (for her, child's pose, with my hand on her sacrum) to make the fear manageable. In trauma work, this way of making manageable by alternating a little time in the difficult place with a lot of recovery time in the safe one is called 'titration'. As Bebe expressed her fear and kept meeting it in small, digestible chunks, it gradually diminished, and she eventually became a confident, skilful headstander. More importantly, she had integrated a fear that originated in experiences as an asylum-seeker fleeing a situation of danger. If my approach had been too cautious, Bebe would not have had the opportunity to encounter her traumatic feelings. If I had been too pushy, too fast, too cavalier, or had not allowed time to be with and listen to her, she might have been overwhelmed by her fear and abandoned *sirsasana* for good, and with it an opportunity for resolving some of her trauma.

We tend to think about safety and risk as opposites, but in reality, it's experiencing sufficient safety that enables us to feel settled and supported enough to move into the scary places in a gradual and measured way. Ashtanga vinyasa teacher Angela Jamison, who blogs as Insideowl, points up the inherent paradox involved in creating safety for transformation:

> [Safe space] is needed for a subversive reason – not to ensure we never feel uncomfortable, but to empower us to go to places of intense internal discomfort without external distraction.[4]

Creating safety for your students is not about being risk-averse or overly protective of them. Yoga teacher Ceri says:

> I went to a class where the teacher actually seemed scared of yoga and appeared to think that most of the postures were dangerous. It was almost as if no one was allowed to feel any stretch or try anything new. We all know that students sometimes want to try things they're not ready for and we need to take them there slowly, in stages, but I'm not the kind of yogi who flings herself around. It was very frustrating.

While we never want to push our students into doing things they don't feel physically and emotionally ready for, we also don't want to collude with their fear. Once trust is established, most people will appreciate the offer of simple, graduated steps to expand their repertoire for moving and being in their body. Mark for the person how and where their capacity has increased – don't silently move the goal posts, and don't let them move the goal posts either. Growth is cause for celebration: so celebrate!

REFLECTION

- Have you ever experienced fear in a posture? How did your teachers work with you in relation to this? Was it helpful? Did you feel pushed? Did you feel supported? What did they do right? What could they have done differently? Did you learn anything from working with fear in this posture? Did your relationship with fear change as a result?

- Have you had students who have been afraid of particular movements or postures? How have you worked with them? What was the outcome? Are there other approaches you would like to try?

- Are there ways in which a yoga class can become too 'safe'? What kind of safe is good? What kind of safe might get in the way of people having important experiences?

Full posture or broke

Tom is another student you may recognise from your own student cohort. His natural inclination is to throw himself head-first into every *asana* opportunity. I value his courage and enthusiasm, but it can sometimes be terrifying to witness! When Tom first came to our Mysore room, he was starting to experience some quite intense pain which was preventing him from doing some of the more gymnastic postures he had practised in the past. He had tried pushing through the pain, but – not surprisingly – it had only got worse. He was now frustrated and scared by his loss of physical capacity. All his familiar strategies had failed – which meant he was now ripe for exploring some different ways of doing things.

The task was to slow Tom down enough for him to be able to feel into what was happening in his body. We used *bandha* to work on foundational structure, not just the big three – *mula*, *uddiyana* and *jalandhara* – but the wider network of *bandha* that extends throughout and stabilises the whole body. We identified movements that were under-used and movements that were over-used. We broke gross movements down into smaller components, so that Tom had all the pieces to move into postures he had previously found inaccessible. I also introduced him to a very experienced physiotherapist who identified some more complex imbalances and helped Tom to change some of his movement patterns, and we incorporated the physiotherapy work into his yoga practice. Initially, Tom needed to reel in what he was doing in his practice, and in some ways he experienced this as a loss. It was important for him psychologically to feel he was setting limits in order to make greater gains, and I often articulated the increased capacity that I was teaching towards. This is a work in progress, but over time Tom has experienced a significant lessening of pain and many abandoned postures have come back into his reach. He has become fascinated by the technique of *asana*, and we are curious to see where skill, control and subtlety will take him next.

REFLECTION

- What is your relationship with risk? How does this manifest in your yoga practice? Has your attitude to risk changed as a result of practising yoga? If so, how?

- Have you taught students whose tendency is to hurl themselves into the most gymnastic posture available? How have you worked with this? Did it help? Are there other approaches you might try in future?

Yoga is a transformative practice

A friend of mine, who has been teaching yoga for about 35 years and is also a trainer of teachers, says:

> Yoga is about transformation, and that isn't 'safe'. I tell my students, 'If you want to be safe, don't practise yoga.'

This statement is provocative (deliberately), but it does contain a kernel of truth. When we practise yoga regularly and sincerely, it has the potential to transform our life from the roots up. We may be impelled to change anything and everything, from our diet through to our closest relationships, our job, where we live, and what time we go to bed and get up in the morning. The physical alignment we work with in *uttita trikonasana*, *uttita parsvakonasana*, and so on does not confine itself to the discrete space of the yoga mat. Embodied work has a liquid quality. It seeps and spreads and shows up everywhere. That's kind of the point. Our habitual stance may be exhausting and dysfunctional, but it's also familiar and unthreatening. In life, as on the mat, there is often discomfort, confusion and a sense of disorientation in the process of realignment.

Many people stop practising yoga when they begin to feel the pull to shift position in this way. We have probably all encountered students who were initially enthusiastic about their new practice – and disappeared, never to be seen again, when deeply buried feelings, self-destructive habits and all the usual mental fudges and evasions began to make themselves known. At this point, the honeymoon period is over and we are invited to cut loose or commit.

In ancient times, when a person began to practise yoga, they were fully cogniscent that they were embarking upon a spiritual practice. They were seeking to bring about profound shifts in being. They wanted to change their mind – literally. The intention of most contemporary yoga beginners is usually rather different. Far and away the most common reason newcomers give me for wanting to start yoga is 'to improve my flexibility', with a few wanting to get fitter, and only the occasional person expressing some sort of spiritual desire. The majority of people think of yoga as a stretching class, perhaps with a bit of prancing around if it's 'dynamic', maybe with some nice chanting, and, of course, relaxation – but not too much, because relaxing doesn't burn calories. In this context, it's not really surprising that many people are terrified when yoga starts to do its real work.

The question arises, then, of what can we, as teachers, offer to hold people through the impulses towards transformation that may make themselves felt when they begin to practise yoga? How can we help to make the risk of change feel manageable? I asked a group of seasoned teachers and these were some of their suggestions:

- Honour the student's need to go at their own pace and, if necessary, take a break from yoga.

- If you are aware that significant trauma is emerging for a student, suggest appropriate professionals who can offer therapeutic help.

- Name it in class. Tony says:

  > I try to explain in advance some of the effects yoga can have – for example, crying during *savasana* as an emotional release – so that if a student experiences them, it doesn't come as such a shock. They can see this as part of a process rather than as a specific personal response or problem.

- Create an open and supportive class structure, and be available to students who might want to talk to you about what's happening in their practice. Christine says:

  > I try to be friendly and approachable, both personally and by email/phone. Students often do discuss with me some of the things

they've experienced. I try not to dramatise any of it but to frame their experiences as one more interesting part of the yoga journey.

- If a student approaches you with a challenging experience, refrain from offering advice. Instead, ask them open questions about it, so that they can discover their own answers.

- Assess the needs of your students in terms not only of how physically fit they are but also of what kind of inner work they might be ready for. Don't rush it. Just as you can over-tax people with postures that are too physically challenging, so you can overload them with chanting, meditation and *pranayamas* they are not ready for. Huma says:

> One of the ways I'm handling this with a private client is by doing an assessment of her needs every time she books a new block. At the beginning, she just wanted to be led through a practice. Now she wants a short sequence to do at home. Initially, she was clear she didn't want any meditation – too 'spiritual' – but she is now open to *pranayama*. Her practice is naturally deepening and the focus is shifting.

- Remember that it's not our job to 'fix' our students – there's really nothing that needs fixing. Several teachers mentioned this.

REFLECTION

- Have you experienced transitions and transformations as a result of your yoga practice? Have you ever felt scared or out of your depth? How did you negotiate these experiences? What helped? Were your teachers aware of what was happening? What was their input? Did you find it helpful?

- Have you ever had to help a student through this kind of transition? What did you do? Was it effective? Are there other approaches you could use in future?

Training to hold securely

J. Brown writes:

> In the training I conduct, I emphasise a set of safety protocols that centre mostly on the teacher–student relationship, scope of practice, and the role that yoga plays in someone's healing and life.[5]

In my experience, though, this approach to teacher training is somewhat unusual. In order to train teachers in this way, trainers themselves need to be proficient in the art of holding a group of students clearly, cohesively and sensitively. In some training programmes it's not unusual for graduates to go straight from the 200-hour course to the 500-hour one, and then immediately to be recruited as course tutors. These trainers have little or no experience of being on the teacher end of a teacher–student relationship or of holding people through the many events that arise in a practice life. Likewise, in the selection process for many teacher trainings, little attention is given to the life experience of applicants. Prerequisites generally centre on attendance at yoga classes (some courses requiring precious little even of that). If you believe that in becoming a yoga teacher you are entering the fitness industry, perhaps none of this matters; if, on the other hand, you understand yoga to be a multi-faceted art and science with the potential to catalyse profound transformations in those who practise it, there's really a very big lacuna here.

So if your teacher training didn't equip you to hold people securely, how can you begin to make up the deficit? In a way, all of this book might be a response to this question, and you will find lots of suggestions throughout. It takes time, practice and intention to cultivate skills in holding people, and however experienced, we are all always practising towards greater capacity in this area. The following are a few key qualities of a teacher skilled at holding a class container. This teacher:

- Holds clear structure and is an effective gardener of the boundaries.

- Is reliable and responsive, and is able to support and include what arises within the class space. It's all grist to the mill of the bigger class plan – the one that they aren't in charge of writing.

- Knows that a healthy class container is a womb-like space; it's strong but it's also elastic. There's room for students to move and stretch and press out the edges, but they also feel securely held.

- Stands squarely in their own feet and is reliable, clear, and responsive rather than reactive.

- Recognises what is in their current capacity to hold and what is not. For example, if they feel scared around people with mental health difficulties, they refer them to a specialist class or teacher. If they feel out of their depth with trauma survivors, they refer them to a trauma specialist. If they feel triggered by the expression of anger, they refer their rageful student to a teacher who is able to stand calmly and clearly before anger.

- Is authentic. They don't assume a 'yoga teacher' persona when they teach; they are present to their students as themselves.

- Listens to their students and respects what their students already know.

- Notices any judgements they are making about why a person is doing a thing and embraces the wide open space of ignorance.

- Refers some questions back to students for their own exploration. They don't themselves have all the answers, and they are honest when they actually don't know.

- Is more engaged in fostering the well-being of individual students and of the group as a whole than in maintaining their own status.

REFLECTION

- What does it feel like for you as a student to be in a safe, effectively held space? Which key skills and qualities contribute to making this space feel both generative and contained?

- Have you ever been a student in a poorly held space? What were the deficits that made it so?

- What does holding an effective space mean to you as a teacher? If you have teacher training, do you feel that it prepared you well to hold space? What was helpful? Where do you need more input?

Scope of practice

While yoga can be a tool for developing the physical body, most (though by no means all) teachers see yoga as far larger in scope and intention, regarding it as an exploration, a life journey, an open question, a passage to different ways of being, an act of presence. Yoga teacher Jemima House says:

> Scope of practice is infinite, encompassing all aspects of living. I'm here to hold space and question in order to guide people towards and through moments of epiphany so their default level of awareness increases. That's one way of putting it. The other is I'm a transition guide, leading by example.[6]

Despite the breadth of this scope, however, one of the many paradoxes of yoga is that intrinsic to its practice is engagement with a physical body that has an anatomy and physiology, and which is subject to injuries and ailments. As yoga teachers, we are bound to negotiate the physiological realities of our students' bodies in an ethical way, educating ourselves about how human bodies work and about which kinds of movement are going to be helpful/ not helpful for common health conditions, and knowing where the limits of our knowledge lie and referring where we have reached them.

For more on scope of practice, see Chapter 4.

Safety in mixed ability classes

I recently started a yoga class for all levels. Three of the women who come regularly find the class very difficult. If we do something like a gentle sun salutation, they get exhausted and often just lie down on their mats. They are so nice and say that they really appreciate the class, but I've ended up teaching very gentle sequences to accommodate them, and they're still finding it hard to keep up. Some of the other students are now getting bored and want something faster and more challenging.

Isla

The general, all-level class is the one-size-fits-all garment of the yoga world, and probably the most common type of class. No wonder. Most small studios and independent teachers lack the number of bums on mats to create different class levels other than the occasional beginners course, and gym-goers often attend whichever class fits into their schedule. If your class is a gentle somatic exploration, or a meditation in which only very simple movement is involved, then you will probably be able to include most people without a problem. If, however, you are teaching vinyasa flow or a reasonably challenging form of hatha yoga, safely including a wide range of people is a lot more tricky. What can you do to make a mixed-level class as beneficial to the widest range of students and as safe as possible?

- Offer a range of versions of each posture and explain to your students that different variations will be appropriate to different individuals. Avoid framing one of these as the destination posture; they are all just alternatives. For more on this, see Chapter 3, 'There is no "peak" pose'.

- Teach to the middle, not to the out-liers. If you try too hard to accommodate the student who really wants to practise 'advanced' postures, the rest of your class will quickly become disenchanted and possibly injured. If you gear your whole class to including the person with chronic fatigue, your other students will get bored and frustrated and eventually vote with their feet.

- Teach to the real capacity of your students, not to a fantasy class. I observe many classes that are way too fast and physically difficult for the people in them, and I receive many students in the Mysore room who have been flowing through sequences of movement with little idea of how to actually do them in a beneficial way. A good teacher teaches in detail, breaking movement down into component parts. Make sure students know what they should be doing and why they should be doing it. If you don't know yourself, don't teach it.

- Move around the room offering one-to-one help and adjustment to students, pointing individuals towards appropriate modifications.

- Refer students who cannot safely be accommodated in your class or who find it over-taxing or too difficult. You are not failing or rejecting the student; you are helping them to find a setting where they can practise without risk of injury and in the most beneficial way possible. This is professional and ethical. Be mindful in your communication with the student, avoiding any implication that they are 'not good enough' to do your class or in some other way inadequate.

- Refer students who want to be challenged more than is feasible in your class. These students need a teacher who is skilled at teaching difficult *asana* in a safe, structured and contained way. If ambitious students are left to go solo in a class not designed for demanding technical work, they may injure themselves in an attempt to produce an approximation of a posture they have seen somewhere but not really understood.

REFLECTION

- Do you teach general or all-level classes? How has this worked for you? Have you had to refer students? How do you manage the different levels within your class?

Serving people with injuries and health conditions

Except in a few instances, yoga teachers are not doctors, physiotherapists or orthopaedic consultants, but many of our students do appear to regard us as medics, with an in-depth knowledge of a wide range of injuries, ailments and genetic conditions. There are, of course, some very experienced teachers who are skilled at working beyond the usual remit of a yoga class. They may be therapeutically trained and may bring to their work bodies of knowledge that lie both inside and outside conventional medicine. But what about the rest? I wondered what sort of training and background yoga teachers as a whole have in anatomy and physiology (A&P), and in working with injuries and conditions.

In a straw poll, I asked yoga teachers about their initial teacher training and about additional trainings they had done since. Around 60 teachers responded, ranging from newly qualified to those with 10-plus years of teaching experience. The amount of time given over to A&P in initial training was hugely variable, with the maximum being more than 60 hours, and the minimum one hour, with the teacher told to supplement by looking on YouTube! At the top end, one teacher commented:

> I got quite a bit of anatomy on my training, plus a test that two surgeons I knew thought was hard!

Another said:

> My entire teacher training course was based on functional anatomy. Every weekend we had at least six hours spread across actual anatomy teaching, discussing *asana* for specific body areas (every weekend dedicated to a different part) and then teaching and adjusting accordingly, first on ourselves, then on the students who came in for two classes every weekend.

Several teachers had received 50 hours – the standard on the British Wheel of Yoga's old diploma. The majority of teachers had received 14 to 20 hours of A&P training, and most thought that this was inadequate. Of these teachers, one already had an additional 180 hours as part of a massage therapy qualification; another was a nurse and so already had pre-existing in-depth training. Several teachers had received only seven hours of A&P, which all considered not sufficient. Many of these teachers had done additional training. One completed a 10-month A&P programme 'almost as long as my teacher training'. The teacher with only one hour of A&P on her initial teacher training went on to supplement it with 20 hours of dedicated training.

There was a similar range of experiences when it came to working with common health conditions, with some teachers (notably several British Wheel of Yoga trained ones, and one trained in Dru Yoga) feeling that they were well equipped to include students with injuries and conditions in their classes. 'It seemed like most of the time was devoted to this – a lot anyway', said one British Wheel of Yoga teacher. Other teachers felt that they were woefully unprepared in this area. One of them said:

> I would have to say information about health conditions was minimal. When I did Thai yoga massage training, we were given contraindications for every pose; it would be so useful to have this on a yoga teacher training.

Most of these teachers were taking supplementary trainings to fill in the gaps.

It's worth pointing out here that training isn't the be all and end all. Of the few golden oldies in this sample – teachers who came up in a time when it was not unusual to learn to teach on the job – several said that they had acquired a wide range of skills and a lot of knowledge, mostly through practical experience. I count myself in this camp. When I started teaching, I had a couple of decades of personal practice, a yoga therapy training and two short adjustment trainings. I was probably a pretty mediocre teacher, but if you keep on keeping on, with consistency and curiosity, it's difficult not to become skilled and knowledgeable eventually. My real area of interest is in emotional/psychological work, but over the years I have acquired a lot of practical experience of working with disk issues, sciatica, knee problems, wrist pain, pregancy and post-pregnancy...and many more conditions. Among old-school teachers, this is often the case.

Setting parameters for safety

Two friends have asked if they can join one of my general-level vinyasa flow yoga classes. One is 58, a beginner, and has a heart condition. She's looking for something that isn't cardiovascular. The other has fibromyalgia and fatigue. She has done a bit of yoga. I don't want to turn them away, but I really don't know if I can include them. My class is quite dynamic and aerobic. I'm worried they will feel excluded if I offer them a private class.

Mireille

When is it safe to include someone with a medical condition in your yoga class? Unfortunately, there's no one-size-fits-all formula for making the call, but there are some basic questions you can ask to get an idea of whether you have the resources in a class to include students with extra medical, physical or other needs:

1. What kind of setting are you teaching in? Is it a big gym class, with different students attending every time? Is it a small class you organise yourself, in which most people attend regularly and you develop relationships with your students?

2. What style of yoga do you teach? Is it fast-flowing, allowing you little time to give personalised modifications or to look at individual students' biomechanics? Is it slow, with each posture broken down and plenty of opportunities for individual work?

3. How experienced is the student and how embodied are they? Are they able to take in and apply a suggested modification quickly, or do they need a lot of time and help to understand it and feel it in their body?

4. How experienced are you as a teacher? Are you a new teacher whose attention and energy are completely taken up simply by creating and holding the class? Are you an experienced teacher, able to keep many balls in the air at the same time?

5. Do you know enough about the condition to suggest appropriate modifications and to know when the student may be putting themselves at risk?

6. Is it feasible for the student to do one-to-one classes with you instead of a group class? Could they do an initial one-off private class in which you assess them, teach them some basics and show them modifications before they – perhaps – join the group class?

7. Is there a suitable class/teacher in your area you can refer the student to?

It's not only okay, it's also ethical and in the best interests of the student to refer them to another teacher if you feel that they will not be well served in your own class – and it's a great idea to get to know the teachers in your local area (or in your gym or studio) and find out what sort of classes they teach and any specialisms they have. For example, a student with a pinched

THE YOGA TEACHER MENTOR

lumbar disc is going to need a slow class with a teacher experienced in back issues; if you allow them to do your fast vinyasa flow class with lots of sun salutations, it's only going to be a matter of time before their back pain worsens and, in the worst-case scenario, they rupture the disc. Even if they really like you. Even if they really like the style of yoga you teach. On the whole, if you are a newly graduated 200-hour teacher with no other relevant training, you are qualified to work with healthy, reasonably fit students with no particular injuries or conditions. If a person does not fit into this category, refer them.

It's important to remember that as yoga teachers, we do not have the tools to diagnose. While experience may give us an idea of what a person's pain or discomfort may indicate, it's only ever that – an idea. For a diagnosis, the person needs to consult an appropriate professional. Be clear about this with students. Don't be afraid of telling them that their question about their dodgy knee/wrist/shoulder is outside your scope of knowledge and experience as a yoga teacher. This will not make you look stupid; it will make you look professional, ethical and well boundaried. For example:

> Question: One of my students has told me that after the class the left side of her neck is painful and she gets shooting pains down her arm. They keep her awake at night and then wear off the next day. I've only been teaching yoga for about a year, and I have no idea what this could be or what she should do about it. Help!

> Response to student: Thanks for telling me. It's possible that this is due to the way you are doing the postures; however, I'm a recently qualified teacher and I don't have the knowledge to understand what's happening. You might want to make a one-to-one appointment with X yoga teacher, who is very experienced and specialises in biomechanical issues. I'd suggest you also go and see your GP, just to rule out any medical causes. Please let me know what you find out. You're welcome to come back to my class once we understand what's happening and know how to work with it.

> Question: A student in my yin yoga class says she feels sick and dizzy whenever we do front-opening or shoulder-opening postures like reclined butterfly. She does other types of yoga and has never experienced this. What is wrong? Why is she feeling like this?

> Response to student: Thanks for telling me. What you're asking me is a medical question, and I don't know the answer. There are many things

that could be causing you to feel like this: you could be dehydrated, you could have a heart condition, you could be experiencing the release of old trauma, or the cause could be something completely different. I suggest that initially you go to see your GP to rule out any medical conditions. It might also be a good idea to talk to X. He is an experienced yoga therapist and can let you know whether this is something he would be able to work with.

Question: One of my students has intense pain in almost all back bends. She thinks she did too much back-bending in the past. I've tried cueing her to use *bandha*, ensuring she isn't putting too much emphasis in the lumbar spine, and making sure her knees and feet are hip-distance apart, but it hasn't made any difference. What should I advise her?

Response to student: We've tried a lot of the standard things that can help with discomfort in a back bend. At this point, there isn't much more that, as a yoga teacher, I can suggest to you. I think it would be a good idea for you to see a physiotherapist so that you can get a proper diagnosis and some guidance about what kind of movements you should be doing at the moment. If you like, I can give you the contact details of a good physio. Please share with me what she says, so that we can take it into your yoga practice.

REFLECTION

- Have you ever tried to incorporate a student with a health condition into a group class and subsequently wished you hadn't? What went wrong? How did you deal with the situation? What do you think might have better served the student?

- Have you ever successfully integrated a student with a health condition into a group class? What factors made it work? What (if any) were the gains for the student?

Serving people with mental illness

I teach a general yoga class in a leisure centre. GPs tend to refer people with mental health issues here because the classes are low-cost.

The problem is, I sometimes feel out of my depth with these students. I don't have any specialist mental health training, and I'm not sure how to keep them safe or if there are things I should be avoiding.

Jay

Mental illness is a portmanteau term for a wide range of difficulties and conditions, each of which has different contraindications and requires different modifications. Broadly, though, we can organise mental health conditions into two categories in terms of how we approach them in a yoga class: depression and anxiety, and paranoid conditions.

Depression and anxiety

People with depressive illness and anxiety conditions can, on the whole, safely participate in all aspects of yoga. A growing number of studies – of a wide range of yoga practices – suggest that yoga can modulate excessive stress responses and decrease physiological arousal, and therefore offers many benefits for people who are depressed or anxious.[7]

Paranoid conditions

People with paranoid conditions (such as schizophrenia or delusional disorders) have also been shown to benefit from the practice of yoga,[8] but more caution is needed here – some yoga practices can make paranoia worse. As a general rule, avoid:

- Sitting meditation.

- Visualisation.

- *Pranayama* other than simply following naturally arising breath.

- Use of belts (which may act as a trauma trigger for those who have been restrained in the past).

- Unexpected or unnegotiated physical contact.

- Use of essential oils or other sensory stimulants.

Stick to *asana* work and provide plenty of grounding and orientation to the here and now – feet on the floor, body on the mat, breath moving in and out. If a student appears to be out of touch with reality, it can help to have them notice what they can see around them – ask them to tell you: 'I can see a patch of light on a blue wall...a green lampshade above my head...purple trousers...' Dina, a yoga teacher who specialises in working with mental health issues, suggests:

> Ensure that the student has their GP's approval to practise yoga. Be sure to set your own boundaries, because co-dependency can become an issue with these students. Ground yourself well before each class and keep track of your energy while you are teaching. It can help to have some sort of grounding and releasing ritual that you do after the class too.

If you feel out of your depth, don't flounder on. Both you and your student can quickly end up in deep water. Explain the situation to your manager if you work in a gym, studio or leisure centre. If you run your own classes, remember that it's professional, ethical and best practice to refer a student to someone with more relevant experience when you cannot safely and competently teach them.

REFLECTION

■ Have you ever taught someone with a mental illness? What worked with this student? What did not work? Are there things that you would do differently next time?

■ What was it like for you to teach this student? Did you notice any changes in your mood, emotions or energy level while you were working with them? How did you maintain healthy boundaries? Did you experience any difficulties with this?

Suspected eating disorders

I teach in gyms and am very aware of girls who are more than usually thin in my yoga classes. One in particular seems to be getting thinner by the week. She looks too fragile to live. I suspect that some students have eating disorders and are using yoga and other exercise classes to help keep their weight down, often attending many classes each week, including dynamic forms of yoga. How should I respond to this student? I don't want to make things worse, but I'm very concerned for her.

Marjie

Eating disorders are very prevalent in our culture, affecting not only young women but also cutting across ages and genders, so the likelihood is that there is always someone with food issues in your class. Because the bodies of eating-disordered people can be any size (including completely average), and eating-disordered people may mask very effectively, on the whole you are not going to be aware that a person has eating difficulties unless they disclose them to you. The students who usually come to our attention are those who are very thin and obviously over-exercising, and the question of how we can be with, teach and serve them in a positive way arises frequently in mentor groups.

As with all our students, the most important thing we can offer a person with an eating disorder is relationship. This doesn't mean being their friend or going out for coffee with them; the relationship in this situation is the profound and transformative one of teacher–student. What we can do for our student in this context is:

- Listen.

- Witness.

- Be comfortable and at home in the present reality of our own body.

- Embody qualities of self-acceptance, self-compassion and kindness.

- Offer honest reflection, if asked for.

Yoga can be part of an eating-disordered person's strategy for weight loss, or it can be a positive influence, or a bit of both, with its function shifting and changing as the person moves through different stages in their relationship with food, themselves and their body. When you are working with someone with an eating difficulty, you will be called upon to hold the tension between the potentially healthful and helpful aspects of yoga practice and the potentially harmful, and to address this sensitively in your teaching, for example, by articulating that in yoga the intention is to feel into and find ways to inhabit our body rather than to improve or transcend it.

It's important that the person knows the teacher is not trying to take their managing behaviour with exercise away from them, but at the same time that the teacher is clearly in charge of what happens in the class – so if the teacher says three sun salutations, they mean three, and no one does five. This creates a sense of strong containment in which it may gradually become safe for the student to relax. Bear in mind that although the eating disorder appears (and in some senses *is*) destructive, it may also be the only thing keeping the person together and alive.

If you feel that you have established trust with the student, this may be a basis for talking to them, from the point of view of an ally, someone who wants the best for them and is willing to listen and trying to understand. Yoga teachers often worry about trespassing in therapist territory – and having appropriate boundaries here is important – however, you don't have to be a therapist to talk to your students, just a human being.

Be aware that it's easy to be drawn into inadvertent complicity with a person who is controlling their life through starving and exercising. This can happen, for example, when we accept a version of reality fed to us by the person, even though it is patently not accurate – for example, that three dynamic classes back-to-back is not really all that many, or that they are naturally 5 foot 10, and 6 stone. To avoid responding in a way that normalises behaviour which is not functional or healthy, my suggestion is that you always speak simply to reality:

Teacher: I see from the sign-in sheet that you've already done four classes today. That's more than I would recommend.

Student: I need to build up strength. My muscles are very weak. It's really important that I do lots of classes.

Teacher: In order to build up strength, your body needs plenty of rest time, and it needs to be well nourished. Extra calories are necessary to create new muscle. Have you thought about pairing a dynamic class with a restorative one?

There is a slow-growing awareness in mental health and related fields that many people with eating disorders are also autistic (and often hypermobile) and are using the eating behaviour as a way of managing a huge amount of overwhelm and distress that they are not able to identify and name. After 46 years of eating disorders, my own food issues gradually ebbed away following an autism diagnosis – which explained intense difficulties I had experienced all my life and enabled me to find more effective strategies to cope with them.[9]

Two good resources for yoga and eating disorders are 'My Big Fat Secret', a short video about how ashtanga vinyasa helped London practitioner Kelly Field with a life-long eating disorder[10] and 'Starved for Connection: Healing Anorexia through Yoga' by Chelsea Roff, the founder of Eat, Breathe, Thrive, a non-profit organisation that helps individuals recover from disordered eating.[11]

REFLECTION

- Have you ever used yoga or other exercise classes to control your weight? Or do you do this now? Has it ever become a problem? Did you find something in yoga classes that was different from classes aimed purely at fitness? Did yoga help you? How? And if it didn't help you, what were the reasons for that?

- Have you had people in your classes who you thought might have an eating disorder? How did you respond? Was your response helpful? What feelings did the situation bring up for you? Are there ways in which you might respond differently in the future?

A therapeutic practice or a risky one?

While some people continue to view all yoga in all circumstances as entirely therapeutic, others speak to the potential risks of some forms of yoga practice. One trend in the current discourse about safety in yoga (fuelled by the infamous *New York Times* article, 'How yoga can wreck your body', published in 2012)[12] is around longer and more rigorous anatomy and physiology training for teachers. On the other hand, some feel that this kind of training shuts down our capacity for tuning in to the body and emerging functional movement patterns from a more somatic perspective. Yoga teacher and movement specialist Amy Matthews says:

> If studying anatomy helps to illuminate the incredible number of 'right' ways to do an action, terrific. Unfortunately, the study of anatomy can also become an imposition of limitations on possibility in a search for what is 'anatomically correct'.[13]

Some feel that the health and safety orientation of modern yoga has bred a climate of anxiety. Elder yoga teacher Jude Murray comments:

> I think this anxiety is partly a feature of yoga training. I meet so many new teachers who are afraid to teach because of the emphasis on injury. Add into that a growing fixation on anatomy. It has its place of course, but I'm not convinced it makes for better yoga teachers.[14]

Indeed, some yoga teachers do feel that they are skating on thin ice as a result of their training. Shona, a teacher in a mentor group, said:

I'm beginning to feel anxious about being responsible for the safety of my students. I've been teaching for a few years now and have really enjoyed it. However, as I gain more experience and knowledge about how to manage different physical issues in class, I've started to feel burdened. I've read a lot about contraindications and feel that all this knowledge is making me too cautious. I emphasise to students that they shouldn't push themselves or do anything that feels wrong, but I'm still terrified that someone will injure themselves in my class. I'm worried both for their well-being and also for my reputation as a teacher.

Minimising the possibility of injury in your class

While it is impossible – and perhaps undesirable – to completely eliminate the potential for injury in a yoga class, there are some simple steps you can take to ensure that your teaching practice is as low-risk for injury as it can be:

- Make sure you have as full a history of the student as possible – and that the conversation about your students' health and well-being is ongoing. Don't expect students to tell you all at the outset. Most people will disclose gradually, as they develop a relationship of trust with you. There's more about student history forms in Chapter 2.

- Teach several versions of each posture and steer away from the 'peak' pose (see Chapter 3, 'There is no "peak" pose').

- Have basic props available – blocks and belts are staples. Be proactive in offering props to individual students where you think they may be helpful. Students often don't have the experience to know when their biomechanics would be aided by the addition of a prop, even if you have explained this to the class as a whole. Show them how they should use the prop and what it is intended to enable, and make sure that they have understood before you move on.

- Check in with individuals as you move around the class. If you know they have a problem knee, when you're passing by ask them, 'How does your knee feel in this posture?' Be ready to respond if necessary with biomechanical cues, props, modifications or alternative postures.

- If a student appears to be struggling or in discomfort, ask them what they're experiencing. If they are, indeed, having difficulties, offer them cues, props or modifications to make the posture more available to them. Don't assume that a suggestion has resolved the issue; check with the student whether it has helped to make the posture accessible for them. If it hasn't and you are out of other ideas, offer alternative postures.

- If you feel that a student is out of their depth in your class, consider whether they would be better served by a referral to another class or teacher, or to a one-to-one session.

- Invite feedback from students on what they are experiencing in postures. Listen and respond to this in your work with the student, especially (but not only) if you are working hands-on. Be in continuing dialogue with your students.

- Check in verbally with students before you adjust: 'Would you like to be adjusted in this posture today?' Also look, feel and intuit what is going on. Does the person's body feel resistant even though they have asked verbally for the adjustment? Be aware that students sometimes feel that saying yes to an adjustment will please the teacher. Make sure you ask about adjustments in an open way, and if necessary, articulate for the student that you really want to know what they would prefer. For more information, see Chapter 4, 'Touch'.

- When you are adjusting, listen not only with your ears but also with your hands. Listen to the whole person, not just to their biomechanics.

- Create a classroom culture in which students' experiences are valued more highly than your own beliefs about what is 'correct' or what 'should' be happening in a particular posture.

- Create a classroom culture in which students feel able to report discomfort or difficulty and ask for modifications, and in which awareness of embodied experience is valued more highly than achieving a particular physical form.

- If you don't know, be clear about this with the student. There's no shame in lacking the knowledge or experience to work with a particular injury or condition. Refer your student to a specialist teacher or other professional who can help.

- Make sure you have a first aid kit in your space. I also always have arnica ointment, Rescue Remedy® and ice packs. These have actually been used in my classes far more frequently than the contents of the official first aid kit. I think the only thing we've ever used from that is plasters. Make sure you have plenty of those.

Responding to injury in your class

A good teacher does their best to work towards the well-being of their students, but none of us has control of outcomes. If we teach out of fear of student injury, we are going to feel constrained and will be limited in what we offer. Students of a fearful teacher may become unrealistically scared of postures themselves, or they may end up feeling frustrated – and may even respond by practising in a riskier way. It's wise to accept that while no one wants a student to be injured in their class, realistically at some point one of your students will sustain some kind of injury. It's not a disaster if this happens. Injury and mishap are part of the learning process, and most often the person will take the set-back in their stride. So when an injury happens, how should you respond?

- Be kind, calm, practical and proactive.

- Don't blame the student and don't apologise to them (except in the rare situation in which you are directly responsible for their injury).

- If the student is more distressed than physically injured, it may be helpful to use some touch: a hand on their sacrum or on their back, for example. Child's pose is a calming posture for many people (but not all, so check first), and you can sit quietly with the person, maintaining a little body contact if they want it. I have done this in a group class and continued to teach while sitting on the floor. If physical touch is not wanted, sitting quietly in close proximity to the person may be welcomed.

- Defuse any drama or excessive sympathy from other students by re-orienting them to their practice. Unless an injury is serious and needs urgent attention, keep the rest of the class in process.

- If an injury has been serious – for example, someone has had to leave the class or an ambulance has been called – devote the rest of the time to helping the group to integrate the experience. If a lot of energy has been created, they may need to jump and shout for a few minutes, or they may need to ground themselves with some floor-based restorative postures – or first one and then the other. You could end by holding hands and sending healing energy to the injured person.

Do what you feel is needed – don't carry on regardless, marching everyone through the class plan!

- Follow up with the injured person a day or two later, asking after them and wishing them a speedy recovery.

REFLECTION

▨ Have you ever felt anxious about your students' safety? Were your concerns realistic? What do you think fed into your anxiety? If you have regained your confidence, how did you do this? Was it a shift in your perspective, or did you take concrete measures to decrease risk?

▨ What does 'safety' mean to you in the context of a yoga class? Is it about following lists of contraindications and precautions or is it something else? Does knowledge of anatomy and physiology make a teacher safer? How do you create a sense of safety in your classes?

▨ Has anyone ever been injured in your class? How did you respond? How were you left feeling after the class? Did you make any changes in your teaching practice as a result? Would you respond similarly or differently to a class injury in future?

'Listen to your body'

'Listen to your body' is a go-to aphorism for many yoga teachers. Yoga is a practice of somatic attention, and so, of course, we do want our students to be open to the word-less communication of the body. However, beware of offering 'listen to your body' as a guard against all injury and mishap. Many injury processes are silent and gradual, and no amount of listening will alert the person to the fact that they are happening. Even when an injury is sudden, it often arrives without prior somatic warning. Working from a body-centred, attention-based orientation does not absolve the teacher from having appropriate knowledge of biomechanics and the capacity to observe their students and understand something of what may be happening in their movement patterns.

While it's true that, as senior yoga teacher Gregor Maehle says, 'The student's body is connected via their nervous system to the student's brain and not the teacher's'[15] – and so a safe teacher does not override the student's experience with their own ideas about what should be happening – it's also the case that many students lack the relevant knowledge and experience to make sense of what they are feeling in their body or to assess where a reasonable 'edge' might be. A safe teacher offers the student sensitive, informed guidance in this. The intention for the teacher is to listen to the student's responses and help them to contextualise these within a framework of what is safe enough and normal experience in a yoga practice. The emphasis is on listening and giving the decision-making repeatedly back to the student, while suggesting where they may want to be a little more outward-looking and exploratory in their approach, or a little more sensitive and self-nurturing.

Teaching when infectious, and infectious students

Nowadays, I rarely catch anything, but there was a time when my immune function was drastically lowered. I spent six months of every year recovering from the flu or prostrate with it, and during that time I was effectively unable to work. The moral of this story is that your minor cold may be someone else's serious illness. And even if it's only their minor cold, they probably don't want it. If you have any illness that your students might catch, it's ethical to cancel your class or get cover – or, if possible, inform all your students in advance that you will be teaching with whichever lurgy, so that they can choose whether or not to attend.

In our culture, many people find self-care difficult and respond to illness by trooping on stalwartly. The greatest service you can do for your students if you don't feel well enough to teach is to model the capacity to honour your need for rest and recovery by taking time off. For some, this can be a powerful teaching.

Likewise, if a student asks you whether they can attend a class while ill with something infectious, the answer is no. You need to look after the well-being of your class as a whole. Direct the student towards a gentle restorative home practice, with lots of bolsters and blankets. There are plenty of practices like this on YouTube.

Boundaries of time

An important part of holding a strong, safe container for your students is starting and finishing on time – right on time. Start and end times are part of the agreement you have made with your students. A safe teacher demonstrates in practical ways that they are reliable and that they remember and honour what has been agreed. You may feel as if you're giving your students something extra by running five minutes over, but actually you are taking something much more important away. Remember, some of your students may have to get away on the dot to be at work or to pick up children. They have entrusted you with the responsibility for making sure they can do that. Take the responsibility. Then they can let go of clock-watching and give themselves over completely to their practice.

A good teacher doesn't get carried away by the momentum of their own class. Remember to track yourself. Inexperienced teachers often try to cram too much into a class, under-estimating how much time it takes to teach a posture or a sequence properly. The result is that students feel rushed or overloaded, and the very important closing and slowing down sections of the class are skimped.

If you teach in a studio or other shared space, keeping good time boundaries is also respectful of the time and professionalism of the next teacher in. If you want good working relationships and the support of your colleagues, don't steal their time! If there's no one else wanting the space after you, and you do feel it would be helpful to run over – perhaps because some incident or other caused a late start – re-negotiate the time boundary with your students: 'Is it a problem for anyone if we finish 10 minutes later today?' If anyone can't stay, then finish at the regular time, even if the person who needs to leave on time says they don't mind. That way you will avoid a ragged ending, with people creeping out at different points, and you will be ensuring that everyone can participate equally.

REFLECTION

▦ Do you always end your classes on time? What helps you to do this? If not, what gets in the way?

▦ If you have a neurological difference such as dyspraxia, time-keeping may be more difficult for you; if this is the case, are there any strategies you use to compensate? If you don't already have time-keeping strategies, can you create some? Are there resources you can draw on to help you – people, books, videos, websites?

The naming of parts

Are there any non-embarrassing ways to teach mula bandha? *I was referring to 'pelvic floor', but then a student asked me what that actually was, and I was literally lost for words. I can't bring myself to say the 'v' word or the 'a' word out loud. Are there any alternatives?*

Margaret

Our classes are inhabited by people with variously one or two breasts, a cock, an anus, a clitoris, testicles, a vagina, pubic hair... If we're not comfortable talking about these body parts, our students will not be comfortable either, and they will not feel that all their body is welcome in the yoga room. Articulating all parts clearly and confidently is central to creating spaces where people can be present whole. Sticking to a few 'safe' words constricts the space and limits of what can be felt and expressed there. If you find it hard to think about genitalia or relate to your own, you may need to do some exploratory or therapeutic work for yourself. If the problem is just saying the words out loud, try walking round the house singing or shouting words you're embarrassed to say, until they cease to trigger a reaction. This idea was suggested to me by several teachers in mentor groups. It worked for them. Avoid nursery words and other euphemisms – they send a message of shame and taboo. Just call a spade a spade.

It's generally best to articulate openly and honestly what's actually happening in the body during specific practices, or what may be. Deep and subtle work with *mula bandha* – the pelvic floor – will most likely elicit a plethora of sensations, some of them sexual. It's helpful to name this aspect of body experience in your teaching and acknowledge that various feelings may arise in response (pleasure, shame, not knowing if what's happening is okay, and so on). Be aware that for students with sexual or birth trauma, bringing attention to the pelvic floor may be difficult, painful or impossible. Provide plenty of opportunities to shift attention elsewhere (for the duration of the exploration, if necessary), and speak to the whole range of possible experiences, both the pleasurable and the challenging ones. This normalises and gives permission for everything to be okay and present in the room.

Breasts, packers and male genitalia

In one class, in which I was, not unusually, the only man, I pointed out to the (young, female) teacher that I couldn't do what she was asking because my genitals were in the way. She went bright red, laughed nervously and walked away.

Ian (yoga teacher)

People in yoga classes have variously lumpy body parts that need to be accommodated in *asana*. Just as we would modify for short arms in a bind, we need to be able create feasible ways for students to enter a posture where they may be obstructed by large breasts or a penis. The more straightforward you are in addressing these challenges, the less embarrassed everyone will be, and the more able to speak up about any difficulties they may be having in working with the particularities of their own body.

Be mindful also of potential difficulties for trans students who pack. When I mentioned packers in a yoga teacher mentor group recently, it emerged that many teachers didn't know what I was talking about, so... A packer is a prosthetic penis worn by some trans people to create a bulge. Some packers are commercially made, include a scrotum and look life-like; others are a rolled up sock. 'Will my packer fall out?' can be a real anxiety for some trans people, and you may need to be sensitive about postures that pose that risk.

Be aware that you may not know you have trans students in your class. While some trans people are obviously gender-divergent, others easily pass as one or the other binary gender and may have chosen not to come out to you. So assume that packing – and binding (breasts to create a flat chest) – may possibly be occurring in your class and teach accordingly. The point is that we never know who is in our class and what relationship individual students may have to our own assumed norms. More on that – and on working with trans students – in Chapter 7.

Taboo body functions

I have a student who is slightly incontinent. I've noticed that when she rolls up her mat – one of my studio mats – after practice, it sometimes has wet patches on it, and so does her bolster. It's definitely urine; I can smell it. So far, I've just been cleaning the equipment, but this won't work long-term. What should I do? I'd hate to make my student feel uncomfortable.

Omid

Yoga bodies may be radiant, but they also shit, menstruate, snore and fart, and generally have the capacity for a wide range of body functions. Lots of these are messy, and they also tend to be somewhat taboo. In situations like Omid's, I suggest that you just talk to your student in a clear simple way about what's happening. I also tend to be a bit stress incontinent in certain situations. I'm not embarrassed by this and speak about it if it's relevant. It's just a normal occurrence that happens in human bodies. In older people, unmanaged incontinence may go with the beginnings of memory loss or dementia, and they may not be fully aware of what's happening. A conversation may highlight the need for diagnosis and support.

The pelvic floor is complex and it's important to be aware that while urinary incontinence can in some instances be due to laxity there (and helped by pelvic floor strengthening), in others the issue is actually hypertonicity, and strengthening will only make matters worse. For referral, a women's health physio would be able to help. A good resource for more information and training on pelvic floor health is Iyengar yoga teacher Leslie Howard.[16]

REFLECTION

▪ Have you ever not spoken about an element of a posture, a *bandha* or some other aspect of yoga because you were embarrassed to use particular words? How do you think this affected your classroom container? How might you be able to articulate this lost and unspoken information in future?

▪ Have you encountered situations in which you needed to speak to a student about a potentially embarrassing body matter: body odour, snoring during relaxation, and so on? How did you communicate? Did the conversation go well? What worked and what didn't?

Death, suicide and loss

If you have been teaching yoga for any length of time, you will probably have experienced death within your student body. In times of grief and loss, most students, even very secular ones, will look to you as a yoga teacher for something more than just an exercise routine. In settings where there is more anonymity and less connection, a death may not be so keenly felt, and a few words of appreciation and sadness at the end of class may be all that's required to mark the passing. But where a group is knit into community, in which members know one another well, attention needs to be given to the process of grieving and of picking up stitches again when the loss has been mourned. You may need to address the feelings, questions and processes surrounding death within your teaching, and to hold strong emotions as they arise for individuals during classes. It can be helpful to create a special event to remember the person who has died, with time to share stories about them, music and poems they loved, food, conversation, dance, and so on.

When a student death is due to suicide it can be more difficult to process, both for you as the teacher and for others in the class. Sometimes the person will have been obviously vulnerable and/or mentally ill, and you may have done everything possible to help – listening, referring, offering an unconditional space for them to be. At other times suicide can be a total shock. You may have had no idea that this particular student was at risk. In the aftermath, you may have to address students' questions about the effectiveness of yoga practice if it couldn't help this individual, and you may also need to attend to your own doubts about what you offered your student, whether it was appropriate, whether you could have done more and so on. In a reflection on losing a student/trainee to suicide, yoga teacher Karen Miscall-Bannon says:

> I think that we all failed. We failed as a community. We failed to create a place for her where she could be real. She was a bright light, always bubbly, and her classes were fun and inspiring to her students. No one saw her shadow side.[17]

This is where sessions with a good supervisor/mentor or Phoenix Rising yoga therapist can be worth their weight in gold. It's essential that you prioritise space for your own emotions and inner explorations at this time. You can't hold a safe and coherent space for questioning and grieving students without it. Remember the resource you already have in your own practice and know that you can modify it. This may or may not be the time for a fast and furious vinyasa flow. Grief lives in the body, not the mind, and embodied practice is necessary to process it. Yoga teacher Seane Corn says:

> After my father died, the grief was so overwhelming that I would become hyper-reactive or numb. I realized you can't just process heartbreak in your mind. You have to process it physically, too.[18]

REFLECTION

- Have you ever experienced a death in your student community? What were the circumstances? How did you help your community to process the event? How did the community help you? What worked? What didn't? What might you do differently next time?

- Have you ever lost a student to suicide? What was your emotional response? How did you grieve and move on? How did you help your student community to process the loss? What worked? What didn't? What might you do differently in future?

EXPERIENTIAL EXPLORATION: SAFE SPACE

You will need:

- Some writing paper and a pen.

- A quiet space where you won't be interrupted for 30 minutes or so.

1. Prepare by entering the terrain of your body through physical movement - see suggestions for how to do this in Chapter 1.

2. Think of a place where you have felt safe at some time in your life, or where you feel safe in the present. If you can't think of one, imagine it. Take your time. This is the kind of safe place where you feel free to create, explore and be. There's no sense of constrainment or limitation here. If this place is associated with a person, you may want to include them too. For example, if your safe place is Grandad's workshop, you can include Grandad.

3. In your imagination, enter this place. Notice what it looks like. Be as specific and detailed as possible in your observation. Are there particular colours, shapes or lines? Can you hear any sounds in this place? Are there tastes or textures? How do you feel here? What do you do? Take your time to fully enter and explore. Give yourself at least five minutes, but you can spend more time here if you like.

4. Now take five minutes to write about your safe place. Do this without stopping, thinking or censoring yourself. If you can't think of anything else to write, keep writing, 'Can't think of anything else to write' until something comes. Don't worry about whether what you're writing is relevant or whether it makes sense. Allow your unconscious mind to guide the process.

5. Read through what you have written once. Then read through it again, this time circling or underlining anything that particularly speaks to you of the nature of this place and what you experienced or experience here. For example, 'Grandad hummed quietly under his

breath while he worked' or 'Lulled by the movement of the waves' or 'A deep sense of peace'.

6. Read through the parts of your writing you have marked. From these, choose six sentences or phrases that feel particularly important to you. Write them down in a list.

7. Look at your list. Notice whether the essence of each thing on it is present in any way in the yoga classes you teach. Be broad and allow connections to suggest themselves. For example, 'Rocking movements on the floor at the beginning of my classes remind me of the lulling movement of the waves', or 'Aunty Jean always listened to me and took what I said seriously; I bring this attitude to my relationship with my students'. Do this with a neutral attitude: don't beat yourself up; don't congratulate yourself. Just notice where there are connections.

8. Mark for yourself any aspects of your safe space that are missing from your classes. Reflect on how you might be able to cultivate them there. You don't need to find answers now. Let the question roll and resonate in your mind and be open to any suggestions that arise.

9. Take time to ground yourself before you return to your everyday life. Notice where you are now and what's around. You may want to have a cup of tea, eat some chocolate, or smell some flowers or essential oils to help you to come back completely to the here and now.

6

The Art of Relating (or 'I Have a Difficult Student')

In some ways, teaching yoga is like parenting. This is not to say that our students are children (unless, of course, they are), but that as the teacher we are responsible for holding the situation, for creating a safe container and being the adult – even when we feel that someone in it is behaving badly. That we will be triggered by our students from time to time is a given. Teaching is a practice in and of itself, which means that at some point every piece of the psycho-emotional junk in our closet is bound to come tumbling out.

Going towards

When we're experiencing difficulty with a person, it's natural and human to want to move away. We may create distance by not adjusting the person, not greeting them or speaking to them at the end of the class, communicating with them by email rather than in person, and so on. One of my teachers, Andrea Juhan[1] (who has been teaching conscious dance and training conscious dance teachers for over 30 years), suggests that when difficulty arises with a student, we actually need to find a way to go towards them.

One of the most powerful ways to go towards is simply physical: we wait for a moment when we feel relatively grounded and centred, and visit the person's space in the room. The intention is not to make the person behave better, or conform to a way we'd like them to be, or do a posture in the way we feel they should be doing it. It's just to hang out with them for a few moments – to receive them, in a spirit of curiosity, and note any somatic information we pick up: for example, 'When I'm near this person I feel angry/sad/hot/cold/distressed/confused'. This information is about us, but it may also offer important clues to what the student is experiencing. While it's important not to project our own feelings and sensations onto a student, it's safe to say that if your general mood is positive but when you enter the student's space you feel overcome by sadness, this is an indication of something the student is experiencing. Making this physical approach may in itself be enough to create a shift in the relationship dynamic, or it may suggest some other way that you might change how you are being in order to be able to accompany this person more effectively in their practice.

Yoga teacher Donna Farhi[2] (another practitioner and teacher trainer of more than three decades) refers to the movement towards as 'the yoga of vulnerability',[3] because entering another person's space naked like this – without assumption, or the need to be seen in a certain way, or the wish to make something happen – requires us to take a risk. We have no idea how we will be met, and we go on in acceptance of that. We are willing to allow the student's response to be legitimate and to be theirs – we don't take it personally. Donna notes that when confronted by someone she finds difficult, she often initially spends a few days just witnessing her own aversions and projections in relation to them. This is important because our first impulse in this situation is often to shore ourselves up in the wrongness of the other person's behaviour and the rightness of our own stance. In order to enter their space empty, however, we have to allow these kinds of self-fortifying thoughts to loosen. Rather than hardening around our own view, we melt a little. We become a little fluid – so that we are responsive and available to receive another person's experience and perspective.

REFLECTION

- Is there a student you have experienced – or are experiencing – difficulty with? What did/do you feel when you are around this person? Let your body respond as well as your mind.

- Do aspects of this person remind you of aspects of yourself that you find difficult to be present to? Or aspects of someone else in your life, for example, a parent, ex-partner, friend, teacher?

- Did you/are you noticing yourself creating distance between yourself and this student?

- What is it like to imagine yourself making an approach of some kind towards this student? (Note that you do not have to actually make this approach if it feels like more than you can handle, or you don't feel ready.)

Isolation and exclusion

Donna Farhi notes that when a 'difficult' person is in one of her teaching spaces, she often becomes aware that the assistants have stepped back from them, leaving them in isolation. She offers this example:

> I am remembering a student with severe scoliosis who was very unpleasant to my teaching assistants and to everyone in the group: like having a stinging wasp in the room! A few days into the intensive I asked her whether she would like to explore a new way of being in her body and when she gave me permission to enter into that inquiry with her, I said, 'I can see that you have been very challenged by your spine. It must be very difficult to live in a spine such as yours.' Within minutes, this angry, bristling bundle of tension, dissolved into tears, and the curtain came down for us to enter into a very warm and productive exchange. She became like a tender child again.[4]

It's not uncommon for other students to step back too, excluding the 'difficult' student from conversation before and after the class, and from any post-class activities, such as going for a coffee. Sometimes students will even gang up and seek to ostracise a student. Maria, a teacher participating in one of my mentor groups, described how this happened in one of her classes:

> I have a student in one of my vinyasa flow classes who likes to 'do her own thing'. She's very flexible and will always be in some sort of extreme 'advanced' version of any posture I teach. The other students have got really fed up with her showing off. They've even asked me if I can tell her to leave the group.

This is a very clear example of a situation in which no one in the class is being held. As she talked more, Maria noted that she often wondered if she was 'too liberal' in her teaching, whether she 'let people get away with doing anything'. Sometimes when she taught a technical point she would see that no one in the class had taken it on board, but she felt uncomfortable about adjusting or verbally cueing the students back towards the teaching she had offered.

When a student is diverging from the 'choreography' of the class, the first response as a teacher is to notice our own reactions: there will often be irritation, projection and judgement there. It's human. Our minds work like this. If we can peacefully greet – rather than suppress or reject – the normal reactivity arising, it becomes easier to re-centre in the teacher place, which is one not of outrage but of service to the student. The second response is to witness the student. Although it can, by the by, elicit a lot of useful information, there's no objective to this witnessing. It's just a way of quietly being with the person – attuning with them. If you have a sense that the student may be receptive, the third response is to enter into an open dialogue with them. This is initiated by asking a question based on something you're seeing. It's important that the question arises not out of the need to make a point but out of the desire to serve in the most effective way possible. If you're still feeling it for the point-making, you're not ready to ask yet. An opening question might be: 'Is your knee comfortable in this position?', or 'What sort of edge are you feeling here?', or 'Would you like some help with this posture?' There's an infinite number of questions because there's an infinite number of students in an infinite number of situations. You ask the question that feels kind, helpful and relevant. Based on this interaction, you and the student may be able start an exploration together.

Mainly, you're seeking opportunities to listen and to collaborate. You don't know why a student is practising in a way that looks show-offy to you. They may be in pain, they may be exhausted, they may be bored/scared/angry. They may be feeling uncontained and pushing to see if they can find a boundary. They may be having difficulty learning the sequence, or they may have missed some of the places where they can find the challenge in it. The student who introduces unelicited 'more advanced' versions of postures is often hypermobile and dyspraxic, and is therefore receiving limited information about how much they are stretching, where their body is in space and how that relates to the positioning that has been cued by the teacher. This is a physiological deficit, not a part of their personality. If the student is also autistic (as a significant proportion of hypermobile and dyspraxic people are),[5] they may also be limited in their capacity to 'read' the effect they are having on other people in the group.[6]

In the mentor group we used role-play to look at some practical ways Maria could keep the class moving and, at the same time, clearly and steadily adjust the off-piste student in a way that enabled her to find the boundaries of her own body, of the posture on offer, and of the class. In doing this, Maria was holding structure for the student in a basic, kind, unforceful physical way. We also discussed why the students in Maria's class might appreciate reinforcement of her teaching with individual adjustment and repeated explanation and cueing – if people weren't doing what she had taught, it might be that they hadn't understood and needed help to integrate it. By making these kinds of interventions, Maria was not being dictatorial but was demonstrating to the class that she was holding the container and looking after what happened inside it. The class could therefore become a safer, more settled space for the students.

When the mentor group met again, a month later, Maria reported that she had found a new authority in her teaching from stepping in and affirming what she was inviting her students to do. The students were delighted and felt that they were learning a lot more in her class. The 'difficult' student had expressed appreciation for Maria's new input. She appeared to Maria more embodied. She was able to follow the form of the postures on offer more closely, seemed more 'with' the class energetically, and was noticing that she felt stronger. There had been no more requests that she be asked to leave the class.

REFLECTION

■ Have you ever had a student like Maria's in your class? How did you handle the situation? Did you feel that the outcome was positive? Are there ways you might want to look after this kind of situation differently in the future?

Holding boundaries: the third way

Maria had a core belief that holding boundaries was something to do with making people follow directions. This is a not uncommon view – lots of us went to schools with a do-as-you're-told ethos. This belief produces a binary in which freedom is equated with absence of boundaries, and everyone can do what the hell they want. In actuality, boundaries function in a third way that stands beyond this binary. A strong, clear, expansive structure creates a safe space for the people in it to explore, ask questions, take measured risks, and express feelings and preferences. In this kind of structure, it's safe to be yourself. Our students want secure but elastic holding, in which there is permission, but there is also containment. When we we are able to be this kind of container, we are serving their needs.

Whose attitude is it anyway?

Whenever I hear someone – one of my mentees or another teacher – refer to 'a difficult student', I wince. In part because I know I've probably often been seen as that student, but also because for me this statement expresses an abnegation of responsibility. A key aspect of the teacher role is being the one who holds the difficulty. When a person in our class presents us with a challenge to relationship, it's our responsibility – not theirs – to breathe, feel and find the space where something can transform creatively. If you feel tempted to describe a student as 'difficult', my suggestion is that you pause, reflect and turn it around: 'I am having difficulty with this student'. This shifting of the onus is crucial and powerful. Your student is just being your student. You are the one having difficulty. It's about you.

Sean brought this experience to online mentoring:

> I had a difficult student on my retreat. I don't mind if people modify postures because they're injured or there's something they can't do, but it wasn't that. The guy told me he had done a teacher training course, but his alignment was all over the place and he seemed to have no understanding of the basics. I tried to correct him, but he just ignored me, so in the end I left him alone and focused on students who were more willing to learn. Was that the right thing to do? Should I have insisted that he do what I was teaching or was I right to let him get on with it however he wanted to?

The language Sean used to describe the interaction between himself and the student was striking to me: 'difficult student', 'correct him', 'he just ignored me', 'students who were more willing to learn', 'insisted', 'let him get on with it'. It spoke to me of a polarisation in Sean's thinking about the teacher–student relationship in which the teacher directs and purveys the 'correct' information, and the 'good' student responds by taking on the teacher's view and doing what they say. I asked Sean how it would be if he considered teaching as a shared exploration in which the student held some information and the teacher held some other information, and they shook it all up together to see what emerged. A few days later, Sean wrote to me:

> When I really thought about it, I realised that underneath, I'm not all that confident as a yoga teacher. I'm quite recently qualified and I rely on the rules I've been taught about alignment. When someone comes into my class with a different background and different rules, I suppose I'm confused, but it makes me want to impose my rules on them. I think in this case, that antagonised the student and made him want to completely ignore me. Maybe I could have found out more about his approach to yoga and seen if there was some way I could work with that.

Outside the window of tolerance

The window of tolerance is a term used in trauma work to refer to the experiential space we are able to inhabit with full, easy presence. There may be challenges within this space, but we are able to meet them adequately and process our feelings about them. When we operate beyond our window, we move into either fight/flight mode (for example, becoming rigid, obsessed, impulsive or resorting to addictive behaviours) or into freeze mode (disconnected, depressed or shut down). The window of tolerance is different for each of us, and for each of us it may be different in different moments and in different situations. For those of us who are are engaged in practices of awareness, it's likely that over the years our window will gradually expand.

We all, at times in our teaching life, encounter students in relationship with whom we are not able to stay within our window of tolerance, and it's healthy to be able to recognise when this has happened. In this situation, it's not only okay to refer the student, it's necessary – from the point of view of your own and the student's well-being. Explain to the student that you feel you are not the right teacher for them at present and that you think they would do better with this teacher, or in that teaching situation. Don't backtrack. Don't waffle. Be kind, be clear and be firm.

Students with developmental trauma

A significant proportion of the students we perceive as 'difficult' in our classes will be the survivors of serious developmental trauma – ongoing early trauma such as neglect, or physical, emotional and/or sexual abuse. When trauma is thorough-going and happens very early in a person's life (sometimes starting before birth), it has profound effects on their neurology and their capacity to formulate an effective sense of self. A person who has not experienced unconditional love, a safe environment or secure boundaries as a child will have immense difficulty in understanding, believing in and identifying these things as an adult. The force of the trauma often causes them to reconstitute the traumatic events around themselves again and again – so if you are teaching a person with a traumatic history, you may find yourself cast in a series of roles that seem to have little to do with who you actually are and how you are relating to the student. These may include abuser, idealised mother, or even victim (with the person believing that they have done something awful to harm you). One of my Phoenix Rising yoga therapy colleagues offered this experience:

> Tom was one of my Phoenix Rising clients, so I already knew he had a history
> of profound trauma when he joined a group yoga class. Before he left each

class, he would always tell me, usually more than once, what a brilliant, inspiring teacher, and wonderful, nurturing person I was. These affirmations were uninvited and inaccurate, and I felt that they were thrust upon me. Any disavowal of them, however, was to Tom just proof of how modest and self-deprecating I was.

Tom continued attending the class for a few weeks, never failing to praise me disproportionately at the end. Then he stopped coming. A few weeks later, I received an email from Tom, asking if he could carry over classes he hadn't used in his block-booking. It was stated in the terms and conditions that block-booked classes weren't transferable, so I explained to Tom that unfortunately this wasn't possible. (Because Tom had developmental trauma, I was aware of the need to uphold particularly clear boundaries with him.)

Tom replied that he felt hurt and disillusioned. 'I thought you were such a kind person, but now I see it's all about money for you.' I responded that in order for our work to be effective, we needed to be clear about the exchange we were making and the boundaries we were setting around it, and that Tom was very welcome to come back to the class at any time. A week passed. I then received another email from Tom: 'I'm so sorry I hurt your feelings. I really didn't intend to. I don't know why I was so horrible to you. You're such a lovely person. I've been really mean. I'm so sorry.'

When a profoundly traumatised student is in your class, you may have a sense that they are not in their body. Traumatised people have often learnt to make this separation in order to protect themselves from physical, emotional or psychological pain. Sexual abuse survivors, for example, may describe how they floated out of their body and watched the abuse from the ceiling as if it was happening to someone else. Traumatised people may not be able to feel basic sensations or to follow simple body-related cues. They may breathe in a stilted way and be unable to relax. They may appear like a rabbit in the headlights, frozen and unable to run. One student who experienced developmental trauma describes it like this:

My muscles are constantly tight, and I can't relax them. It's as if I have to be always ready – whether there's any actual threat present or not. This means that I suffer constant pain. Because I sometimes stop myself from breathing, I suffer panic attacks. Paying attention to my body is terrifying, because memories of abuse come up. I am really shy within a group and scared to give my opinion.

It's beyond the scope of this book to offer a protocol for teaching yoga to traumatised people. Several have already been created – perhaps the best known is the Trauma Center's Trauma Sensitive Yoga (TCTSY).[7] The following are a few general suggestions for avoiding some of the pitfalls that can arise when we attempt to include traumatised people in a general group yoga class.

Hold clear, strong boundaries

Traumatised people have often had little or no experience of appropriate boundaries. By definition, their own most basic personal boundaries have been violated repeatedly. Typically, traumatised students will test every boundary you set – often by what feels like covert means – and will become upset, angry or ashamed if you try to point out to them what they are doing. This is because on a volitional level, they did not set out to transgress. Remember that trauma is operating on a neurobiological level. The tugging and pulling at the limits is happening outside their conscious awareness and control. As a result of their dysphoria around boundaries, these students have often ended up in abusive adult relationships with teachers and therapists. You will best serve traumatised students, yourself and your other students by clearly stating and simply insisting on basic boundaries. Don't be tempted to make any exceptions. For any reason.

Be a safe person for the student in class

A traumatised person may have a pronounced startle reflex and may appear jumpy. Don't approach them suddenly. Let them see you coming and give them time to acclimatise to your presence. Be mindful about physical adjustments – but don't assume that a student with trauma won't want them either. This is a place for sensitive dialogue. Be aware that some traumatised people cannot give meaningful consent because they have been conditioned to consent to everything and feel that they have no choice. Be slow and gradual with any agreed touch, and use your intuitive and animal senses to feel into whether the person really wants it, regardless of what they are saying. Re-check with them often and encourage them to give you verbal feedback on how they are experiencing the adjustment – in a way that acknowledges their power to change it: 'Is this too strong, just about right or not strong enough?' 'Would you like me to stop?' 'Would you prefer not to be adjusted at the moment?'

Don't take it personally

A traumatised person is, to a greater or lesser degree, a captive of their past experience and is continually replaying the past in the present. This may blinker them to what you are actually saying and doing. Their tendency will be to fit you into a limited repertoire of known roles from their past. When they can no longer square the circle of who you are with the role in which they've cast you, they may catapult you into a different one. This dynamic is happening on a neurological and somatic level, and this is where resolution needs to happen. The person cannot change their beliefs or behaviour by thinking about them and rationalising, or by trying. The most helpful way to be with this is to remain completely neutral, letting the student's projections slide off you like the proverbial water off a duck's back. This is, of course, a lot more difficult than it sounds. Subconsciously, the traumatised student is constantly trying to hook you into their drama, and they will be very good at this. Expect to feel alternately protective, insensed, afraid, compassionate, confused and more when you are interacting with a student with trauma. Know that this is not about you, or about the student, but about the way that trauma impacts upon a human being and how they relate with others.

Refer appropriately

If you are over your edge, it's ethical to tell the student that you feel you are not the appropriate person to teach them. Make yourself aware of trauma yoga teachers offering classes in your area, and of somatic therapists, yoga therapists and body-based psychotherapists with a specialism in working with developmental trauma, so that you can have some referral suggestions ready. Ideally, rather than feeling ditched, the student should have a sense that you are concerned about their welfare and guiding them to a place where it can be looked after more effectively. Trauma yoga teachers teach yoga to traumatised people in an appropriate way, but they do not work therapeutically, so you may need to refer the student to a teacher for their yoga practice and to a therapist for deeper, more thorough-going work.

It goes without saying, but let me say it anyway… Your job as a yoga teacher is to teach yoga. Never attempt to address the person's trauma in (or outside) a yoga class. And even if you are trained to work with trauma, do not attempt to do this in a class environment. A class is not a safe or appropriate container for a therapeutic intervention.

Don't be attached

Davina was new to yoga when she joined a restorative yin yoga class, where she was receiving help from an assistant teacher as well as from me. She didn't declare trauma on her student history form, but it was quickly obvious that she was traumatised. She appeared terrified, breathed shallowly, had difficulty identifying simple sensations, and seemed to be floating several inches above her body. She was unnaturally 'cooperative', and it was difficult for us to find out what she was actually experiencing in different physical positions and therefore to know if/how to help her to modify them.

Davina found it difficult to organise props and place herself in a comfortable position, but we kept working slowly and steadily, and she kept coming to the class. One day, I spent some time helping her to place a bolster and blanket in a supported back bend. I left her with the assistant teacher and when I next turned around was startled to see Davina rushing out of the room with tears in her eyes as the assistant teacher looked on, stunned.

When I went out to find out what was happening, Davina said: 'You've been unnecessarily harsh with me. I just don't need this. I came here to learn yoga, not to be told off. I think you're being really strict and it isn't nice.'

I hadn't told Davina off; I had been trying to find out where was comfortable for her and what support she needed. But Davina wasn't experiencing me or my interventions; she was re-living an event from the past and re-construing the meaning it had had for her then around what was happening now.

It's easy to believe that you can be the one to turn things around for a traumatised student – especially when (as often happens at the beginning of the relationship) the student is idealising you and constantly telling you how beneficial they are finding your teaching to be. Yoga and other body-based practices can indeed be very helpful to traumatised people, but trauma is deep-seated, and change usually happens gradually, over a long period of time. It's common for traumatised students to disappear suddenly and unexpectedly. Their lives are often internally and externally turbulent. Their window of tolerance is quite narrow, so they quickly hit the limit of how much they can integrate. Embodiment can be fraught for a person whose only experience of body is rape, violence or humiliation, and even simple and apparently unthreatening embodied practices, such as noticing a sensation or feeling their breath, can trigger traumatic memories for them. Know this, and allow the person to disappear without notice or explanation when they need to, and leave the door open for them to return if and when they're ready.

Be prepared for things to go 'wrong'. It happens – regularly – even to those of us who are experienced at working with trauma. As my own trauma therapy supervisor reminded me, the real work of trauma recovery happens through relationship, and the ordinary trials and tribulations of relating are essential to this process. Know that, as the space-holder, you did your best, and take what may feel like failure in your stride.

REFLECTION

- Do you ask students about PTSD/developmental trauma/history of physical or sexual abuse in your student history form?

- Do you have students who have divulged developmental trauma? Or students who you suspect have experienced developmental trauma? How does the trauma show up in the way they are in your class and how they relate to you?

- Have you experienced any difficulties in working with these students? Notice any physical sensations or strong emotions that arise as you recollect what was difficult. Do these belong to you, or might they be an individual student's experiences?

- Are there ways that you might want to change how you work with these students in future?

Autistic students

Autistic people are another group often perceived as 'difficult' in yoga classes. Autism is a variation in neurological processing style, with a variety of ramifications in terms of the kinds and amounts of different types of information the person receives and how they make sense of it. The needs of autistic people in a general yoga class is a big subject, and I've written about it at greater length elsewhere.[8] Here, I'm going to touch just briefly on some of the main misunderstandings that can occur when an autistic person enters an allistic (not autistic) setting. Be aware that not every autistic person in your class will have a diagnosis or any inkling themselves that they are autistic – autism is still massively under-recognised. And even if they do have a diagnosis, they may choose not to declare it on your class joining form. Autism is still very stigmatised, and many autistic people are closeted.

But autism is also fairly common, and it would be unusual if you never had an autistic person in one of your classes.

Articulate the 'rules'

An autistic person may not pick up the unspoken social rules about how to behave in your class in the way that an allistic person would. So if, for example, an autistic student asks a question in the middle of *savasana*, it's probably not because they are being demanding, but because you told them questions were welcome but didn't say that *savasana* is a silent section of the class. If they place their mat at right-angles to everyone else's, or at the front, next to yours, it's less likely that they are showing off or trying to be disruptive and more likely that you have not explained that all the mats should be level with each other and parallel, with the short end facing the front. 'Everyone else is doing it like that' may not strike an autistic person as a good reason to do it like that too. We tend to do things in original ways.

Be aware that even if the autistic person in your class appears to be socially adroit, they aren't. Some of us are adept at imitating others and using learnt scripts to fake social intelligence. This method is not foolproof, and we often get it, if not totally wrong, then a bit off-kilter. Those autistic people who 'pass' in this way are perhaps the most at risk of being branded 'difficult' rather than seen simply as lacking capacity to 'read' socially.

Liza told me:

> In my big classes, I have teaching assistants. They usually practise along with the class until I need them. In one class, I gave the nod to my assistant, Morag, and she got up and went over to help a student who was struggling to keep up with the sequences. I quickly saw that things weren't going well between them. The student didn't seem to be taking on board what Morag was saying and was more or less ignoring her. Afterwards, Morag said she was really rude and uncooperative and didn't seem interested in learning anything. I decided to investigate, and the next time the student was in the class, I asked her whether it had been helpful to have an assistant working with her. She looked puzzled. 'You know, when Morag helped you in the last class?' I said. The student went bright red and stared at the floor. Finally, it emerged that she hadn't realised Morag was an assistant. She had thought she was another student who had just started telling her what to do! I later found out that this student was autistic. I now realise that I should have explained to the student that Morag was an assistant rather than assuming she would just get it.

Create a low-sensory environment

Autistic people may be very sensitive to sensory stimulae and can be driven close to the threshhold of sanity by a humming light fitting that you can't even hear, or by the sensation of the carpet, or by a (to you) almost invisible dirty smudge on a wall in their sight line, or by the vestigial smell of incense from a class three days ago. Deirdra, a dynamic vinyasa flow teacher, told me about this experience:

> Part-way into one of my classes, an autistic woman who is a regular student told me she was having difficulty with the body odour of a couple of the people in the class. To be honest, I didn't take this very seriously. I mean, everyone gets sweaty in a dynamic class, and it's something you just have to live with. Anyway, they didn't smell that bad to me. I thought she was being a bit melodramatic. I suggested that she move her mat, helped her relocate it, and didn't think anything more about it. Some way into the class I became aware that she was curled up on her mat. When I went over to find out what was wrong, I realised she was actually retching. The body odour was so intense for her that she was literally nauseated. I didn't know then that autistic people have heightened senses. At the time it all seemed a bit weird, but now it makes total sense.

Auditory sensitivity can combine with verbal processing difficulties, as in this story that Darryl told me. He was teaching a private class for an autistic student in a studio space divided by curtains:

> I was explaining something, and for some reason – I didn't know why – he was looking increasingly distressed. Then he put his hands over his ears and buried his head between his knees. A few moments later, he got up quickly and left the studio. When I found him outside, he explained to me that he couldn't separate my words out from what he could hear other people saying in the other curtained-off spaces. The words had got all jumbled up and he had felt as if his head was going to explode.

For more on working with autistic people, see Chapter 7, 'Neurodiversity'.[9]

REFLECTION

- ▨ Do you ask students about autism and other neurodivergence (ADHD, dyspraxia, dyslexia, etc.) in your class joining form?

- Do you have autistic students or students you think could be autistic? How have you helped them to manage the physical environment and the social expectations of your class?

- Have there been any misunderstandings? Were you able to rectify them in a positive way?

A change of perspective

It's not unusual for a teacher to come for mentoring annoyed because something in their interaction with a student seems to be getting in the way of them actually teaching the student: 'They're resistant and don't want to listen to my instructions'. In my view, this is back-to-front. I see teaching yoga as essentially relational. It may look as if we are teaching postures, alignment and breathing techniques – and these are not unimportant – but they are the structure, not the content. They are a pretext for one human being (the student) to come into relationship with another human being (the teacher) in such a way that the student is offered an opportunity to witness their own emotional, physical and mental tendencies and perhaps change some of them. In fact, this is a two-way process. Our students offer us an opportunity to notice our tendencies too – which is one reason why teaching is also a practice – but for the teacher this is something that happens not in the company of the student but in the alembic of our own reflective space, and perhaps with the help of our own teacher or mentor.

The shift to teaching from this perspective can be transformative. When you work in collaboration with your students, in service to their own process of discovery and with their best interests at heart, you no longer have to be an expert with an answer for everything. Phew! What a relief! You are simply an interested and informed companion, committed to creating conditions in which each person's own authentic embodied intelligence can emerge.

EXPERIENTIAL WORK: BEING A DIFFICULT PERSON

At some point in our life, most of us will have experienced being cast in the role of 'the difficult person'. The intention of this exploration is to pitch yourself into that experience, recollect the feelings and responses that go with it and - hopefully - shift your perspective to one that is inclusive of 'difficult' students, not by an effort of will, but through empathic iden-tification.

You will need:

- Drawing paper, coloured pens, crayons, pencils – or anything else you like to draw with.

- A quiet space where you won't be interrupted for an hour or so.

1. Prepare by entering the terrain of your body through physical movement – see suggestions for how to do this in Chapter 1.

2. Think of a situation in which you were the 'difficult' person for an individual or group of people. If you can't think of any situation in which this happened to you, imagine one. Take some time to remember the place, the time in your life, the feelings aroused and your responses. If at any point remembering becomes overwhelming, step out. Go and do something different. Come back to this exploration when you feel ready – or just leave it for now.

3. You are going to make a drawing about this time called 'The difficult person'. You can approach this in any way you like. Your picture can be figurative or abstract, colourful or black and white, minimal or detailed, big or small. If you like, you can include words. Everything is allowed.

4. When you feel done, step out for five minutes. Go and make yourself a cup of tea or go outside into the fresh air.

5. When you come back, look again at your picture. What do you see? Are there particular shapes or colours? Is there a mood? How have you used the space? What does your picture tell you about what it's like to be considered a 'difficult' person? If emotions arise, allow yourself to feel them fully and then let them move through.

6. Now take a moment to think of a time when you were one of the gang, part of a team or a valued contributor. If you can't remember an experience like this, imagine it – this will be just as powerful. Notice any feelings and physical sensations that arise. Consider the two very different roles you have played, or have imagined playing, in different situations.

7. Resume your day.

7

Including Every Body

In this chapter we will be looking at inclusivity – how do we make our teaching accessible and inviting to all sorts of people? In mentor groups, many teachers are genuinely flabbergasted when I suggest that inclusivity is about more – much more – than being warm and friendly to whoever shows up at our classes. Were this sufficient, the yoga demographic would reflect that of the general population, which, some specialised settings aside, it clearly doesn't. While a small number of teachers are already inclusivity-aware and actively working with under-represented groups, on the whole as a profession we are apathetic when it comes to promoting diversity. Yoga teacher and body positivity advocate Jessamyn Stanley says. 'The more that I travel, the more it nauseates me how inaccessible yoga is.'[1] Strong words, but it takes proactivity to make yoga classes friendly to people who statistically are unlikely to attend them. If we want our yoga spaces to be really inclusive, we have to abandon the rainbows and unicorns 'happy place' fantasy of yoga as exempt from socio-cultural influences and magically available equally to everyone, and begin to take concrete action to widen participation.

This chapter is by no means a comprehensive examination of how marginalisation happens and who it affects, but I hope it will stimulate you to think about groups of people you may unwittingly be excluding from your classes – and about simple ways in which you might be able to make your teaching more available to them.

Tangible barriers

Fortunately, most church halls and community spaces are equipped with lifts, ramps and disabled toilets these days, so a lot of our classes are going to be accessible to people using mobility aids. If your venue is one of these, give disabled people[2] a break by stating this clearly in your publicity. Being disabled entails so much work that people without disabilities don't have to do – particularly where the disability involves the need for a wheelchair or mobility scooter. If you include access information on your website, that's one extra email a disabled person won't have to write. It's just a little bit of strain you can take off their shoulders.

Occasionally, you may need to teach somewhere that isn't wheelchair-accessible. One of my venues, a complementary health centre, is in a Victorian house up a steep, narrow flight of stairs. There's no space in or outside the building for a stair lift or a ramp. I use this venue anyway because it's independently owned and run, and while it isn't accessible to those with mobility needs, it does serve other marginalised groups.

Yoga teachers sometimes believe that their style of yoga is too dynamic to appeal to a wheelchair user and that wheelchair access is therefore not an issue for them. There is no style of yoga that is too dynamic to appeal to a wheelchair user. It's true that some people using mobility aids have conditions that involve fatigue, and are therefore unlikely to be interested in a Rocket Yoga class, but just like those of us who walk on legs, wheelchair users range from the disinclined to do anything energetic to the super-fit and athletic. I've had wheelchair-using participants in a led ashtanga vinyasa class.

Being based in a city, I also make it a point only to use venues that are well served by public transport, and therefore more likely to be accessible to people on a low income. It's more environmentally friendly too.

Toilets and changing facilities

If there are no gender-neutral toilets in your venue, queer and trans people who do not 'pass' as one or other of two binary genders (male/female) may be put off coming to your class. Dealing with potential queer- and transphobia, along with the whole range of potential micro-aggressions around who's allowed to piss where, can feel just too much. These may be people who simply don't experience themselves as either male or female (and therefore are not comfortable in either binary-gendered toilet) or who are in transition and appear out of place in toilets designated for both their assigned-at-birth gender and their gender of identification. Josetta Malcom, a yoga teacher offering classes for the LGBTQ+ community, says:

> Lots of yoga studios have very gendered changing rooms and toilets, so sometimes trans, genderqueer and non-binary people will get very 'policed' and questioned over which changing rooms and toilets they've used.

They may also feel as though they're being judged or looked at in some way. But it's not just trans, genderqueer and non-binary people that get policed in this way. Because some lesbian, gay and bisexual people don't present in the way that mainstream society expects them to, they can be policed too.[3]

According to Jane Fae, lack of appropriate toilets is one reason why historically many trans people have suffered from urinary tract infections: 'hold it until you're back in the safety of your own home'.[4]

If you teach in community spaces, changing facilities that aren't a corner of the room or a toilet cubicle may be a dreamed-of luxury, but if there is a designated changing space, the same issues around who is comfortable using it are going to apply. While access to a physical space is important, perhaps even more so is the message you send out by attending (or not) to questions of toilet and changing room accessibility. If you haven't thought about the toilets, you probably haven't thought much about the whole experience of a queer, trans or gender-fluid person in your class.

REFLECTION

- Are your class spaces wheelchair accessible? Did you have to think before you answered this question? Do you include accessibility information on your publicity? If you haven't thought about any of this before, let go of any guilt or self-blame; just note that it's something you can be aware of in future.

- What kind of toilet and changing facilities are available at your class venues? Might they be excluding certain students? If so, is there anything you can do to improve the situation?

Invisible barriers

If your class spaces aren't equipped for wheelchairs, walking frames and mobility scooters, people who use these aids will not be able to access your classes. That much is pretty easy to understand. But why might an autistic person, a lesbian or a black person experience exclusion from your classes? While very few yoga teachers are actively hostile to members of marginalised groups or fail to welcome them if they do show up at a class, there are often factors at work outside our awareness that create barriers to access for certain groups.

Othering and assuming

If you are a member of a marginalised group, you've probably had the experience of being talked over or about – as if you were a research monkey, an alien, a plague or a moral outrage. As an autistic person, I've lost count of the number of times I've been lectured about myself by an allistic presenter, as if no autistic person could possibly be in the room, because we're all rocking in a corner with our hands over our face and definitely unable to understand a lecture. As autistic writer Rhi says:

> When experts talk about autism – trainers at work, speakers at conferences – they often seem to forget there will be autistic people in the audience. We become 'they'. We are 'othered' by the very people who are supposed to know the most about us.[5]

'Othering' is a particularly horrible experience, provoking feelings of shame, anger and voiceless-ness. Unfortunately, yoga culture is particularly prone to this kind of side-lining and omission. Yoga teacher and social justice activist Dianne Bondy suggests that the reason for this obliviousness is that we have forgotten to practise *svadhyaya*, self-study, the examination of our beliefs and attitudes.[6] Most often insidiously rather than deliberately, we fail to recognise that people with different kinds of bodies, lives, brains and cultural experiences also exist, and that – visibly or invisibly – these people, too, are potentially among our student group.

REFLECTION

- Have you ever had an experience of being 'othered'? What did it feel like? How did you respond? Were you able to advocate for yourself? If you have never had an experience of being 'othered', notice that.

- Have you ever talked over a member of a marginalised group in your teaching? Did they pull you up for it? If so, how did you respond? How did you feel? Notice the physical sensations and emotions that arise as you remember this experience.

Language

For a teacher, language is a key tool. We want to be able to use it effectively to communicate with all our students – that goes equally whether we're languaging through speaking, through writing or through signing. If we're leaving certain people out when we use language, we're not communicating effectively. Trans man and yoga teacher Nick Krieger says:

> I have experienced more instances of hurtful and invisibilising gendered language, assumptions, and jokes than I could possibly mention in a single blog post. Jokes about pregnant men that discount trans men who carry babies. Cues where men do this and women do that, erasing trans folks. Assumptions about the body parts that men have and the body parts that women have when who knows what body parts a person has under their clothes.[7]

Inclusive language enables everyone to feel welcome, valued and invited to contribute. It avoids making assumptions and perpetuating stereotypes about people based on their age, race, sexual orientation, gender, dis/ability, and so on.

Gender

What makes me feel excluded from a yoga class? Being called a 'lady'. It seems trivial, but this is really common when a group is (assumed to be) all female. 'Okay, ladies?' Assumptions about gender make me too irritated to relax into my practice.

Jude Murray (yoga teacher)

Unless they've told you, you don't know how your students gender themselves – even if you think you do. Most people assume from the way I look that I'm a woman, but that's not actually how I identify myself. The handles I use are 'fluid', 'agender' and 'human'. As Jude notes, there's often an 'all girls together' assumption when a female yoga teacher teaches a class that appears (to her) to be all women. Even for those who do gender as female, being thrust into what has suddenly become defined as a women-only space, one in which certain 'female' ways of being and relating are presumed, can feel uncomfortable when that isn't what was signed up for. Unless you actually are teaching a class designated for women only, keep your language inclusive, and don't start rabbiting on about wombs and the special qualities women are presumed to share. Rather than the dreaded 'ladies' (which connotes a set of attitudes and behaviours that alienate even many of those who do gender as female), use neutral words such as 'everyone' or 'people'.

If you're unsure which pronouns to use for a particular person, it's fine to ask. This is a normal question about a normal thing, so don't make a meal out of it. Just say:

What's your preference for pronouns?

Then try to remember – but if you do forget or get confused, just apologise and correct yourself:

I'm sorry, Lex. I meant 'they'.

Getting it right all the time is far less important than showing yourself willing to listen and respect individual gender identities, and being seen to do your best.

Languaging pregnancy yoga classes

> Our pregnancy yoga classes are friendly, fun and relaxing, and a great place to meet others expecting a baby. Birth-givers often make lasting friendships. We welcome all sorts of families, and people of all genders and sexualities.

Wouldn't it be great if queer-friendly advertising like this actually existed for pregnancy yoga classes? I couldn't find any, so I made up this example myself. There can be few places where queer and trans people are more excluded by the language of cis-gendered heteronormativity than in yoga classes for pregnancy. I can vouch for this personally as someone who had a baby within a queer family. If you teach pregnant people, know that:

- Not everyone carrying a baby genders as female.

- Not all families consist of two parents (in some families there are three…or one…or some other number).

- Not all co-parents are in sexual/emotional relationship with each other.

If you are a pregnancy yoga teacher, the chances are that you would have no issue whatsoever with, say, a lesbian birth-giver and her female partner attending your class – but if your publicity refers exclusively to cis-gendered, heterosexual birth-givers, the lesbian soon-to-be parents are unlikely to sign up. Not without reason. If you didn't think about them when you wrote your publicity, it's unlikely that you will be aware of their needs in the holding of the group.

There are plenty of more inclusive alternatives to 'mums', 'mummies' and 'pregnant ladies'. In her article '8 gender-neutral birth terms and how to use them', sexual health expert, doula and alternative therapist Tynan Rhea suggests 'birthing person', 'person in labour', 'co-parent' and 'primary care-giver', among others.[8] Broadening the scope of your language will also make your classes attractive to a wider range of cis-gendered straight women, some of whom may not warm to being referred to as 'mummy' and may feel queasy around some of the more cutesy language that abounds in pregnancy yoga teaching. The key thing is that you talk to individual students and find out which words they use to refer to themselves – and respect their language choices when you address or talk about them. If your student loves being referred to as a 'mummy', great, call them that, but don't make assumptions about what is acceptable to particular indviduals or impose your own language preferences on everyone.

Fat/curvy/large people

On the one hand, a person in a yoga class is just a person in a yoga class, and there's mostly no need to draw attention to different body sizes; on the other hand, there are going to be times – when adapting a physical assist, for example – when fat (as with height, limb length, body length and cleavage) is going to make a difference. Skirting around the obvious just creates awkwardness and prevents effective communication from happening. The great thing is that we can talk to our students and find out their language preferences. Obviously, in the case of a large/curvy/fat person, this requires sensitivity, and we may need to be investigative. Some people (even those whom others would consider to be thin) experience a paralysing amount of shame about the size of their body – and no wonder, given the rigorous policing of fat in our culture. Don't assume that it will be rude to refer to your student as fat. Fat-positive activist Cat Polivoda says:

> 'Fat' is my preferred term. There is an element of reclaiming the word that I love. I think it's easier to actively resist misconceptions about fat people when I am comfortable with using the word. For instance, when people insist that I am 'not fat' but I am, instead, 'beautiful', I can remind them that I am both 'fat and beautiful'.[9]

But also don't assume that they are fat-positive and embrace fat-positive language. It can be helpful to open the conversation by addressing your group as a whole. For example, you might tell your students at the beginning of the class:

> This is a body-positive class. People with all sorts of bodies are welcome: old bodies, young bodies, black bodies, brown bodies, white bodies, able bodies, disabled bodies, thin bodies, fat bodies…and everything in between. Basically, if you're human, you have a place here. If there's any language you do or don't want to be used in relation to your body, please do let me know.

Some words are positive for some people but offend others. I want to respect your preferences in relation to your own body.

Be aware that, as a medical term indicating dysfunction, 'obese' is not a fat-positive word. Neither is 'overweight', because it presupposes that a person's weight is in some undefined way 'too much'. For what? Health, well-being, attracting a partner, getting something to fit in a mainstream clothing store…? Who knows? For a discussion on the languaging of fat as a descriptor, see Ragen Chastain's 'Is it ok to call fat people fat?'[10]

REFLECTION

▨ Have you ever been excluded by a yoga teacher's language choices? How did the experience make you feel? Did you try to talk to the teacher about it? What was the response?

▨ Does any of your habitual teaching language exclude anyone? What words could you use instead? Do you need to check in with anyone about how you address them?

Lack of people who look like you

White teachers don't always notice you're there – that you look different, that yoga is Indian and might mean something else to some south Asian people like me. It's uncomfortable. Sometimes I'm one of two or three Asian students. On my teacher training I was one of two. Now I'm teaching and usually the only person of colour in the room. It's weird.

Nadia (Asian-British yoga teacher)

If you don't see people who look like you doing yoga, it's hard to believe that you have actually been invited to the party. 'I think a lot of us see yoga as something that's not for us, because of the lack of imagery', says black yoga practitioner Robin Rollan.[11] To some extent, the over-representation of white women in yoga practice has to do with the modern history of *asana*. Much of the yoga we practise now has been heavily influenced by fitness and exercise regimes created in the early twentieth century to appeal to young, white American and European women.[12] Many yoga classes – particularly the vinyasa flow forms – continue to be geared towards this group.

Men, not normally considered a marginalised group, are often a minority in yoga settings. When cis male beginners get in touch with me to enquire about a class, it's not unusual for them to ask whether other men take part, what they wear and – essentially – whether, as a man, they will stick out like a sore thumb in the class. The distinctly girly presentation of much popular yoga is a put-off for a wide range of people who are not lithe, young and white, who do not aspire to conventional femininity, and who are looking for something more thorough-going and substantial than rhythmic gymnastics.

Cost

It's difficult to make a small independent yoga studio pay: acknowledged. However, at the time of writing, it costs £17 to do a class at one of the big, established studios in London – more than twice the National Minimum Wage (currently £8.21/hour). When you factor in the cost of travelling to and from the studio, your yoga class is going to come in at well over £20. Big-time studio yoga is clearly affordable only for those with a generous income. While some of the major studios do offer concessions, information about them is, on the whole, difficult to find, and the concessions are generally for students and pensioners, and so miss some of those on the lowest incomes, the waged poor and disabled people without access to benefits – who in most cases can't come to a low-cost community class in the middle of the working day either.[13]

Independent teachers working out of church halls and community centres (ourselves often among the lower paid) are generally charging considerably less, and frequently offering sliding scales, concessions, work exchanges, and so on. Few of us will refuse a student who genuinely wants to practise yoga, even if they can't pay in money. However, we have far less publicity clout than the big studios and tend to be little seen and known. The general impression therefore continues to be that yoga is for rich people.

Sensory barriers

Sensory overwhelm is the number one thing that will stop me going to a class. It may sound trivial, but synthetic smells (deodorants and perfumes) are a barrier. They stop me focusing and sometimes trigger allergies.

Thea (yoga teacher)

Proximity to clothes washed in chemically perfumed detergents and fabric conditioners, music, incense, and even synthetic carpets can act as a barrier to participation for autistic people and others with sensory sensitivities. The gym – with its video screens, fluorescent lights, multiple sources of noise and many people in a small space – is pretty much a no-go area for those with sensory challenges.

Racism, ableism, homo/transphobia inherent in the teachings

There are numerous ways in which traditional teachings, and some contemporary interpretations of them, reflect social prejudices. Paradigms based on *shiva* and *shakti*, 'masculine' and 'feminine' energies, for example, may create an obstacle to participation for the gender-fluid, for whom the notion of an energy having a gender is just perplexing. Accessibility is generally broadened where the teacher maintains an open attitude to yogic, New Age and other philosophies, recognising that each is a system of thought, one among many, rather than a universal truth shared by everyone.

Clothing

> *The kind of fitted and often revealing clothing worn in many yoga classes is a factor in putting some Asian women off. Muslim women are discouraged from wearing clothes that disclose their body shape, and they are often not comfortable dressing in leggings and figure-hugging tops. This is a pity, because older Asian women in particular are often missing out on exercise.*

Ayesha (British-Bangladeshi yoga teacher)

If you come from a background in which fitted and/or skimpy clothing is considered unacceptably sexual…if you feel uncomfortable exposing body parts that look different due to a genetic condition or disability…if you experience body shame or dysmorphia…you may not be comfortable dressing in the crop top and leggings/ripped-torso-revealing yoga shorts that appear on social media to be *de rigueur* in a yoga class. Access can be widened by reassuring students that any comfortable clothing they can move in easily is fine for yoga. Baggy trousers and a long top are perfectly acceptable, and clothing from your local discount retailer will work just as well as branded yoga wear.

REFLECTION

▨ What kind of messages might your own teaching clothes send to your students? Are these the messages that you want to communicate?

▨ Small changes can have significant results in increasing access. Are there things you might easily be able to do to make your classes more inviting to a wider range of people?

All sorts of bodies

All too often, yoga is becoming a phenomenon of the fetishised body, and I think it's our job to guide people away from that.

Frances McCourt (yoga teacher)

Our attitudes towards bodies – both our own and other people's – condition (often silently and without examination) what and who we are able to include – fully – in our classes. Some common assumptions include:

• Fat people are unfit and unhealthy.

• Thin people are fit and healthy.

• Disabilities are visible.

• Very flexible (hypermobile) people do not experience pain when practising yoga.

• Middle-aged and older people are unfit.

Sometimes some of these things may be true, but none of them is a given. The truth is that we can tell precious little about a person's health, fitness and general capacity simply by looking at them.

The average teacher training cohort is composed mostly of young, flexible, thin and generally female bodies; this is therefore the type of body that trainees get to practise teaching. As a result, there may be huge gap in skills and understanding when newly qualified teachers begin to encounter actual students, many of whose bodies are stiff, old, deconditioned, male and/or fat.

Fat bodies

It can be no news to anyone that lean, muscular bodies are valorised in our culture, while fat ones are considered to be unattractive and unhealthy. 'You've lost weight!' is supposed to be a compliment, whereas 'fat' as a descriptor is regarded as tantamount to abusive. In few places is the demonisation of fat more clearly in evidence than in the mainstream yoga world, making a visit to a yoga studio for a fat person potentially intimidating and shaming. Dancer, fat activist and yoga practitioner Ragen Chastain says:

> Many fat people have had terrible experiences at a regular studio, where the teacher assumes they're a beginner, is unwilling to touch them or is condescending and sees them through their own prejudice.[14]

Fitness enthusiast and yoga student Tiffany Kell says:

> Of all the sports and athletics I have participated in as a fat person, yoga has sadly been one of the most judgmental and the least emotionally safe.[15]

So what can we, as teachers, do to create supportive, positive teaching spaces for students with large/curvy/fat bodies?

- Be aware that fat does not automatically equate with unfit. Like thin people, some fat people are couch potatoes while others walk, swim, run and work out.

- Be aware that fat does not automatically equate with unhealthy. The relationship between fat and health is complex and multi-factorial, and a quick Google search will reveal a diversity of opinion on whether being fat compromises wellness.

- Do have the same expectations of fat students that you would of anyone else. Until or unless you discover otherwise, assume that they have similar capacities of strength and endurance, and that they are no more or less flexible than your not-fat students.

- Find opportunities to reinforce for all your students that fatter bodies are potentially no fitter or less flexible than thinner ones.

- Be aware that modifications will often be necessary to accommodate body curves. Work exploratively and collaboratively with individual students to find out what they need, and have a look at some of the online resources on modifying for fat bodies.[16]

- Offer adjustments to your fat students if you offer adjustments to others. As with modifications, work in an exploratory and collaborative way to find out what works – and do your research.

- Express through your language and your actions that there are many different types of body and none is better or worse than another. (This will also be helpful to any students you may have with disordered body image.)

- Find out which words individual students prefer to be used in relation to their body – and use them. (See 'Language' above.)

- Be in dynamic relationship with your own prejudices, preconceptions and attitudes to fat – both in general and in relation to your own body. If you think you don't have any prejudices, think again. We are all surrounded by highly pathological attitudes to fat, and even if you personally have embraced body positivity, it's likely that there will still be subversive voices with less enlightened opinions sounding off in your head. The most helpful response here is to listen: this is good information about our less voluntary and seldom acknowledged thoughts. Then thank the speaker for their contribution and move them aside, well out of ear-shot. What is heard and acknowledged tends to settle of its own accord.

- Know that your attitude towards your fat students can make a huge difference, not just to their yoga practice, but also to their relationship with their body:

  > When I heard my teacher say, 'See what Anna is doing over there? Do it like that'… I'm not sure I've ever had a prouder moment in my life. Someone was shining the spotlight on me for showing up in my body, this body, and doing my thing. This showed me some critical things: that I was capable of being present in my body and responding to it, that being connected to and not hating my body was possible, and that yoga was playing a big part in helping me get there. (Anna Guest-Jelley, yoga teacher and founder of Curvy Yoga)[17]

- Don't assume the person wants (or needs) to lose weight. Jayvin Jordan-Green, a student at Fat Yoga studio, says:

  > I've had teachers who said, 'This is going to help you stay thin' or 'This is going to get rid of this unwanted roll here if we keep practising'.

It's like, 'Maybe I like that roll, maybe the people I date like that roll.' I had a lot of teachers treat me like I'm their special project. They'll say, 'I'm going to make you the buffest person.' They see me as the 'after' picture, when I don't want to be the 'after' picture.[18]

- Don't reinforce negative views of fat bodies.

- Don't assume that because someone is fat they should be in a slow, gentle yoga class.

- Don't refrain from offering help when the person needs it – or assume that the person needs extra help simply because they are fat.

- Don't patronise or sympathise. Fat yogi Jagger Blaec says:

  The one thing I couldn't get used to were the sympathetic stares from the instructors. From the time I walked past the front desk to the end of my practice, the puppy-dog eyes never ceased.[19]

- Don't act embarrassed or shilly-shally around the reality of your student's body. Be straightforward, respectful and proactive in teaching them – just as you would with anyone else.

REFLECTION

▨ Have you ever experienced judgement or discrimination because you are (or have been) fat? Has it ever felt difficult to walk into a yoga class?

▨ What sort of judgements do you make, or have you made, about fat/curvy/large-bodied participants in yoga classes (your own or ones you were a participant in)? Have you ever made assumptions about the fitness/flexibility of a student based on how fat/thin they were?

▨ How do you serve fat/large-bodied students in your class? Are there things you might be able to do to serve them better?

Disabled bodies

One hallmark of a skilful yoga teacher is the capacity to work adaptively. This entails an ability to listen and collaborate, and to create original approaches to meet particular needs. Being able to innovate on the hoof in this way requires a willingness to let go of dogmatic views and think out of the box.

If you are deeply rooted in your own practice and accustomed to working exploratively with what needs accommodating in your own life (injury, pregnancy, burn-out, renewal, and so on) you will already have a solid basis for teaching in this way.

Iyengar yoga teacher Matthew Sanford[20] is one of the pioneers of the adaptive yoga movement. Paralysed from the waist down in a car crash at the age of 13, through the practice of yoga Matthew discovered that while he might not have voluntary movement in his lower body, it was far from 'dead', as he had been led to believe, but rather, was full of subtle energetic movement:

> I can't lift my legs. I can't flex the muscles. But I feel a hum, a tingling, a buzz... The instructions in an *asana* are intended to amplify your connection to that hum... Because of my paralysis, I understand and appreciate that the sound Om is actually calibrated to that buzz, to that hum.[21]

Matthew trains teachers to work adaptively and also teaches a broad spectrum of students, including those with paralysis.

While some disabled people have conditions that involve fatigue and will therefore need a slower, gentler practice, others are fit and active and want to be challenged. If the person is used to working with their body, and to collaborating with a teacher to find ways to make movement sequences accessible, they may be pretty easy to integrate into a regular yoga class. Depending on the style of the class and how much time you have to work with individuals in it, you may also be able to include less experienced students in a general class. Have a look Wanderlust's film, 'Arm Balance: The Practice of a One-Armed Yogi', for an example of how one teacher and his new student made a success of this.[22]

As with all specialist teaching, it's skilful to recognise:

- When you lack the knowledge and experience to include a student with a disablity.

- When your class is not an appropriate setting for meeting particular disability needs.

Refer appropriately. No one expects you to be able to do everything or include every disability in every class.

Inspiration porn and ablesplaining

Those of us who have a disability are accustomed to the expressions of amazement and disbelief that frequently meet any disclosure of doing perfectly ordinary things (tying our shoes, making dinner, walking the dog, practising yoga). My social media feeds are replete with inspirational clickbait involving plucky paraplegics climbing mountains, Deaf[23] dancers, painters with Down's syndrome and all the rest. While it's fantastic that diverse human beings are expressing themselves and reaching their potential, disabled people are not here to astonish and uplift you. We're just getting on with normal stuff, sometimes in creative ways. Disabled yoga teacher Shakti Bell is matter of fact about her ability to teach yoga: 'I usually don't move especially quickly, navigating in a wheelchair or simply crawling to reach students.'[24] Disabled people in your class are likewise just doing yoga. Don't patronise them or make assumptions about their experience of disability by praising their courage, endurance or capacity to overcome.

Also be aware that the person is always the authority about their own experience. Don't try to explain your student's disability to them because you've read up on it or done a course on it. (We call this 'ablesplaining' in the disability activist movement.) Know that they are probably already aware of the information in the fantastic article you've just come across on Facebook, they're not interested in CBD oil, and have already tried changing their diet. They come to your class to do yoga, and your remit as their yoga teacher is to offer them the frameworks, information and holding they need to do that.

REFLECTION

- Do you have a disability? What have your experiences been of accessing yoga classes? What has been helpful? What has not been helpful?

- Have you ever included a yoga practitioner with a disability in one of your group classes? Or worked with a disabled yoga practitioner one-to-one? How was it for you? How do you think it was for them? What did you learn? Would you do it again, and under what conditions?

Neurodiversity

Neurodiversity encompasses dyslexia, dyscalculia, dyspraxia, autism, ADHD, Tourette syndrome and other processing differences. The term 'neurodiversity' implies that there are many natural neurological variations in processing style, each of which brings advantages and challenges, and all of which are essential for the well-being and development of human beings as a species.

In terms of practising yoga, the form of neurodiversity with the most direct impact is probably dyspraxia, a deficit in spacial awareness that involves difficulty in judging our position in space and the spacial relationship of one body part to another. A student with dyspraxia may need to repeat a posture, or a change in body alignment, many more times than a non-dyspraxic student would in order to embody it. Dyspraxic students are often labelled lazy, inattentive or not interested in 'corrections' by teachers who either do not identify the student's dyspraxia or do not understand its implications. A person with dyspraxia requires a patient teacher who is willing to repeat the same adjustment or verbal cue again and again without becoming reactive, understanding that repetition is an essential part of the process of integration for this student.

It's also important to be aware that all the neurodiversities are in a cluster of intersecting conditions that include hypermobility (Ehlers-Danlos syndrome, hypermobility spectrum disorder and so on), and a student with any kind of neurodiversity is fairly likely also to be hypermobile.[25] There's a lot more information about working with both hypermobility and dyspraxia in my article, 'Hypermobility on the yoga mat'.[26]

Unidentified neurodiversity

I have a situation with a student, and I have no idea how to handle it. She arrives 25 minutes before the class starts, when I'm still preparing and not ready to engage with students, but she plonks herself on the mat right in front of me anyway. Sometimes she starts moving the other mats around or turns the heating up or down. She doesn't follow the sequence, ignores instruction and pushes her body way beyond what it's capable of. She's hypermobile and 'hangs' in her joints, but if I try to pull her back or offer a prop, she just ignores me. She loves doing wheel, which I don't teach, and is constantly flinging herself up into it uninvited. If I teach a breath practice or lead a meditation, she zones out, and she leaves during savasana *– sometimes not before she has called someone on her phone and had a conversation with them while still in the room. I've tried dealing with this by talking about* yamas *and* niyamas, *but to no avail. I've told her that I think I may not be the right teacher for her, but she keeps coming to my class.*

Kirsty

Students with neurodiversity are often undiagnosed, unaware of the ways in which their behaviour is at a tangent to accepted norms, and confused about why they are unable to fit in. In yoga class settings where the teacher does not recognise why the student is being the way they are being, they are often stigmatised and labelled as rebellious, unwilling to learn, high-handed, and the like.

The experience in the quotation at the head of this section was brought to a yoga teacher mentor group by a fairly new teacher. The student she described immediately struck me as probably autistic, but in a mentoring setting I always want to hear what everyone else has to say before I put anything into the pot, so I invited the group to respond. I was struck by the blame and judgement that teachers initially directed at Megan's student:

> Her behaviour is disrespectful to you and is disrupting the other students. She has to change it or stop coming to the class.

> That sounds like a pain in the arse. Do you actually want someone like that in your class? Her attitude is rude and selfish.

> She has bad energy and it's affecting everyone else in the class.

> The solution to this is simple. Ban her from the class.

I noticed that Julia, herself autistic, hadn't spoken, and I asked her if she wanted to contribute anything. Tentatively she said:

> I'm wondering whether this person might actually be autistic. I see some autistic traits here.

I asked Julia to tell the group about the traits she had noticed. She pointed out that the student seemed unable to pick up on the teacher's need to be alone at the beginning of the class or to 'get' that it was not socially acceptable to arrive 25 minutes early. She appeared not to be 'reading' the unspoken rules of the yoga class. She was having a lot of difficulty with being still, which is often overwhelming for autistic people, who need to move in order to process the huge amounts of information/stimulae being received from both inside and out. Julia also commented that as a hypermobile person, the student was probably not able to understand experientially how a prop could help her or to feel that she was hyper-extending her joints.

I invited the teachers in the group to shift their perspective on this situation – to consider that this might actually be a teaching relationship in which the teacher was confused about how to hold the student adequately, and to ask themselves what she might be able to do to make her class container larger, clearer and more substantial so that it could also encompass this student, who appeared to be unable to find the boundaries. What might this student need from her teacher? These are some ideas the group came up with:

- Explain the social rules of a yoga class to the student – clearly and kindly. Don't assume that she will automatically understand that it's inappropriate to arrive 25 minutes early or that she is encroaching on the teacher's preparation time.

- Tell the student – clearly and kindly – to come out of the wheel when she goes into it uninvited, and redirect her to the posture the class is working on.

- When offering a prop, explain how it will help the student to create more muscle engagement, to be stronger and more stable in the posture, and to improve her *asana* work. Stay with the student and show her how to use the prop, pointing out where she needs to be working more actively and how she can pattern her body in a more functional way.

- Tell the student evenly, clearly and directly that she may not talk on the phone during the class and explain that this is because it disturbs other students.

- Ask the student about her experience in *savasana*. If necessary, clarify the purpose of *savasana*. Ask her whether there are any adaptations she might need to be able to stay present for this important part of the practice (whether she needs to sit, to keep her eyes open, to have permission to move quietly and unobtrusively). If she feels that *savasana* is really beyond her at this point, negotiate a way for her to leave the room quietly and respectfully beforehand.

- Engage directly with the student about the challenges and deficits that hypermobility involves: talk to her about the difficulty of feeling the end points of an extension and explore ways of feeling more into mid-range. Educate her about the proprioceptive difficulties hypermobile people experience.

- Elucidate the rules. Explain what is allowed and what is not.

For more about working with autistic people, see Chapter 6, 'Autistic students'. See also my article 'Autistic movers and shakers'.[27]

Responding to a challenge by someone from a marginalised group

Imagine this scenario:

> You are a white European teacher. Inspired by an interesting article you read last week, you are talking to your class about the meaning and cultural context of the word *namaste* – while a Hindi-speaking British-Indian student is in the class. The student raises their hand and points out, from first-hand experience, that some of what you have said is not correct.

When a person from a marginalised group speaks out to correct an assumption a teacher has made about them, their culture or the group they belong to, there is an opportunity for communication, education and understanding to happen – if the teacher is open to it. How can you enable a positive outcome? Here are a few suggestions.

- Practise humility, listen respectfully and apologise for talking about someone who was in the room, and whose knowledge of their own culture is deeper and more reliable than yours.

- Ask the person if they would like to tell the class more (but don't expect them to educate you all – it's not their responsibility).

- Know that it takes courage to contradict someone in a position of authority (teacher), and all the more so when you are the only Indian/disabled/gay/other minority person.

- Keep things in proportion. Stay present. Continue to hold the space – by paying attention to and including your student's contribution. A skilful teacher is able to weave in all the threads.

- Know that in helping to dispel the dusty old cobwebs of your *avidya*, the student is doing you a favour.

- Don't get defensive or try to demonise the student ('they are rude/disrespectful'; 'they want to undermine me').

- Don't shrink back in shame, lose yourself in your own emotional responses, or otherwise make it all about you.

For an excellent and very readable article on how to listen to and respect the experiences of disabled people, see 'Listen to our experience: On epistemic invalidation' by Naomi Jacobs.[28] Many of the principles outlined in the article are also transferrable to other marginalised groups.

REFLECTION

■ Have you ever been challenged by a student from a marginalised group? How did you feel? How did you respond? What do you feel in your body as you recall this experience? Is there anything you might want to do differently next time?

Self-advocacy/disclosure of special needs

Self-advocacy is when a person speaks up about about a personal need which is not being met, usually because it is at variance from the needs of the majority and therefore has not been considered. The disclosure of a need might be:

- I need you to use the correct pronouns for me; my pronouns are 'zi', 'zim', 'zir' and 'zis'; I will understand if you make a mistake, but I need you to try.

- I need you to give me modifications appropriate for my body size; I can't do some of the things you suggest because my 'rolls' get in the way.

- I need you to offer me adjustments even though I'm practising in a wheelchair; I still want to work on getting into the postures, and I want to be touched.

- I need you to treat me as one of the crowd; please don't behave as if I'm the only gay in the village or make a joke out of my sexuality.

- I need you to stop using that essential oil because it makes me feel sick.

- I need you to face me when you address the whole class so that I can lip read you.

- I need you to stop referring to me as 'coloured'. If you need to refer to my race, please use 'black' or 'person of colour'.

If we want to expand participation, we have to be open to listening to people who sometimes feel uncomfortable or out of place in yoga classes – fat people, queer people, trans people, disabled people, black people, poor people, working-class people – and making changes to accommodate them, rather than justifying the way we already do things or dismissing their experiences. So how can we respond in a helpful way to a self-advocacy?

- Listen, ask clarifying questions if necessary, and see what you can do practically to meet the person's need.

- Thank the person for speaking up and helping you to understand their needs.

- Allow yourself to be aware of any uncomfortableness you feel – and give yourself time to feel into and unpick this later.

- Be aware that when a person (especially someone from a marginalised group) advocates for themselves, they are making themselves vulnerable; your willingness (or not) to listen and understand can be make or break for your relationship with this student.

- Don't talk over the person.

- Don't try to defend what you already do.

- Don't diminish, minimise or deny the person's experience ('But everyone else loves this essential oil'/'My nextdoor neighbour is fine with me saying "coloured"').

- Don't take it personally – this isn't about you.

When we believe that we are a sensitive and caring teacher who includes and welcomes everyone, self-advocacy by a student who hasn't felt appropriately seen, understood and accommodated can be distressing and may dent our self-image and provoke a crisis of confidence. This is all to the good. Challenge expands our capacity as a container, enabling us to hold a more diverse group of people more fully and safely. See this is as an opportunity to grow, rather than an experience in which you felt ashamed and undermined.

Your intention to listen, learn and accommodate is a lot more important than always getting everything absolutely right (which is impossible anyway). Mia Mingus, who describes herself as 'a disabled Korean transracial and transnational adoptee', has coined the term 'access intimacy' to describe the particular embodied sensation of having your access needs 'got', of feeling that you are not struggling alone but that you are seen, heard and acknowledged in all your humanity, not in spite of but inclusive of your disability. She says:

> [Access intimacy] is not dependent on someone having a political understanding of disability, ableism or access. Some of the people I have experienced the deepest access intimacy with (especially able-bodied people) have had no education or exposure to a political understanding of disability.[29]

I think that 'access intimacy' is translatable to feeling seen, heard and got, not only in terms of disability access needs, but in terms of all forms of marginalisation. We don't have to understand the politics of race/homophobia/body shaming, or know the politically correct language. We just have to be willing to listen, stay present with the messiness of it all, and do our best to relate.

REFLECTION

▦ What special needs do you have in your current student group? How do you go about meeting them? Might there be needs that have not been expressed? How could you invite them into the room?

▦ Have you ever dismissed or ignored a special need? What were the reasons? Would you still respond in the same way?

Expanding the reach of your publicity

If I had a pound for every piece of yoga advertising I've seen featuring a lissom, scantily clad, 20- or 30-something white woman, performing a pretzel posture on a sun-kissed beach… Yes, I'd be rich, right? This kind of publicity picture is so prevalent it's become yoga wallpaper. As social justice activist, accessible yoga teacher and the leader of the Yoga For All movement Diane Bondy says:

> We are in no way offended as we continue to be bombarded with homogeneous images of yoga and the world at large. In fact, most of the time, it doesn't even register in our consciousness how debilitating and detrimental these images are! We are completely unconscious of our actions, our words, and our influences on the people and the environment around us.[30]

While teachers and experienced practitioners may sigh and scroll on by, in the mind of the regular non-yoga-doing population this is the default image of a person who goes to a yoga class – and most of them don't fit it. Exclusion has usually happened long before a student enters your class space; it operates in our minds when we are considering possibilities, framing parameters, constructing habitats in which we may feel we belong.

Who, then, might the yoga wallpaper be excluding?

- People who aren't white.

- People who aren't female, including those who are agender, fluidly gendered, transgendered or intersex.

- Middle-aged and older people.

- Fat people.

- Inflexible and unfit people.

- People from a culture in which scanty clothing is not considered appropriate for women.

- People who can't afford beach holidays in exotic locations.

- Disabled people.

To be clear, if there were only a few images out there of pretzel-on-a-beach woman, none of this would be a problem. There's nothing inherently wrong with being young, flexible and white. The problem is the dearth of images of stiff, black, brown, old, queer, poor and disabled people also doing yoga.

Representing real students

I teach slow, basic hatha yoga. It would be great for older people, but I rarely see anyone over 40 in my classes. How do I attract a more senior group?

Myra

For me, there's nothing duller than a website full of images of a teacher demonstrating postures – except maybe a website full of stock images. From a marketing point of view, this kind of content also flies shy of the target. As a teacher, your product is your capacity to create engaging spaces for others to explore the various facets of yoga, to encourage, catalyse and explain – not your ability to perform *asana*. The other problem with this kind of website is that the only people who see themselves reflected on it are the ones who look like you, so the images drastically limit the site's potential social reach.

A good, easy way to make your website more engaging and to broaden its representivity is to feature images of an actual class: real students, real teaching. Obviously, you can't just start taking photos in your regular classes: it's disruptive of practice space, and you don't have your students' consent.

What you can do is organise a special photo shoot class. Make it clear to your students that a photographer will be present on this occasion (so they can opt themselves in or out), and offer the class free in return for permission to use the resulting images for publicity. If you can afford to pay a professional photographer, that's great, but if money is a problem, which it may be if you're just getting your teaching off the ground, try inviting a good amateur photographer with an interest in photographing movement. Ask around local photography courses and amateur photography groups, and see who your students know. If you want to attract, say, more elderly people to your classes, encourage your existing older students to take part and ask them to invite their older friends. The interested but nervous, who are teetering on the brink but haven't yet tipped over, may be tempted by the free class – and you could gain some permanent students.

It's good practice to ask everyone taking part to sign a release form. I also give everybody the right to veto any pictures of themselves they absolutely hate. No one has ever actually done this, but knowing that they can may be reassuring to some students. Subject to agreement with the photographer, I also offer participants access to any images of themselves for their own personal use.

I've done the class photo shoot several times, and my experience has always been that it stimulates communication between participants, fosters connection and deepens community. People love seeing the photos, sharing them and talking about them, and (an unintended plus) from a technical point of view, they sometimes also learn things from seeing themselves in postures ('I didn't know I did that with my arm in triangle!', 'I never realised my forward bend was so deep!').

If you'd like some inspiration, check out the website of Unfold studio (Portland), which was created to be inclusive of all sorts of bodies and represents a wide range of actual students.[31]

REFLECTION

■ How representative is your publicity of the people who come to your classes? Of the people you would like to attract? Of the population where you teach? Are there changes you'd like to make to encourage different groups of people to attend?

Inclusion and accessibility policy

It's both good practice and inviting to people from marginalised groups to have an inclusion and accessibility policy, and to publish it on your website. This shouldn't be a legalistic document or a disclaimer – which would be the opposite of inviting to people from marginalised groups – and it can be short and sweet. This is mine:

> I do my best to create safe space for people of all ethnicities, sexualities, genders, neurologies and dis/abilities. As an autistic person, I'm aware that what excludes us is often invisible to others, so if there's anything you need in order to have full access to a class, or anything you'd like me to know, please do talk to me – we can work it out together. Most group spaces are wheelchair-accessible: details are on individual class listings. For more information, please get in touch.

Addressing the question of inclusion in itself sends out the message that you are aware of marginalisation, that you want to accommodate people from marginalised groups and that you are open to having a dialogue about what individuals might need in order to access your class. I know that I am far more likely to give an activity a try if there is a clear indication that the facilitator is willing to engage positively in meeting my needs.

EXPERIENTIAL EXPLORATION: BEING IN/BEING OUT

You will need:

- Some writing paper and a pen.

- A quiet space where you won't be interrupted for 40 minutes or so.

1. Prepare by entering the terrain of your body through physical movement - see suggestions for how to do this in Chapter 1.

2. Think about the last time you went to a yoga class. Take some time to imagine yourself back into the class. Where was the class? What was in the studio or class space? What did the teacher look like? Who was there? Which practices did you do?

3. Think about any ways in which there was ease or a sense of belonging for you in the class, ways in which you felt welcome and part of the gang. Write them down. If you didn't feel any sense of belonging, remember or imagine a different occasion (a yoga class or some other

kind of event) at which you did feel at home and one of the group. If you have never experienced this sense of being one of the group, imagine how it would be. Your list might include things like:

i. Lots of students were also young women.

ii. The teacher smiled at me when I walked in.

iii. My body shape was similar to the shape of most other bodies in the room.

iv. Everyone was speaking my first language.

v. The person on the next mat chatted to me at the end of class.

4. How did it feel to have a sense of belonging? To fit in with the group? Notice how your body responds in the present. Include any feelings, sensations and emotions that arise, even if they seem irrelevant or unimportant. Spend a few minutes on this reflection and write down anything that feels significant to you.

5. Now think about any ways in which you did not feel at ease or welcome, or were not sure whether you belonged in the yoga class, and write these down in a new list. If you didn't experience this at all, think of another situation in which you didn't fit in. This could be a different yoga class, or it could be some other event (a job, a party, a group dinner). Your list might include things like:

i. I was much younger than everyone else.

ii. Everyone in the class was white.

iii. Everyone was wearing really expensive-looking branded clothes.

iv. I was the only person with a disability.

v. All the other people seemed to know each other already and no one talked to me.

vi. Everybody was straight, or acted as if they were, and it didn't feel safe to come out.

6. How did it feel to be out of place, to sense that you did not belong and were not fully part of the group? Notice how your body responds in the present. Include any sensations and emotions that arise, even if they

seem irrelevant or unimportant. Spend a few minutes on this reflection and write down anything that feels significant to you.

7. Read through everything you have written: both lists and both sets of responses. Going on these personal reflections, what do you feel are key things that make a person feel welcome and part of a group experience? Write a list of these, elaborating where necessary.

8. Think about your own classes. Bearing in mind what you have learnt about your own experiences of being included and excluded, what do you already do well as a space-holder? And what might you want to do differently in future? Write down any changes you would like to make.

9. Take a few minutes to sit quietly, just noticing any thoughts, feelings, images or sensations that arise.

8

Experienced Teachers

What constitutes an experienced teacher? For me, there's more to it than a catalogue of training and a tally-up of contact time.

An experienced teacher has a body of dedicated practice experience, not classes taken, or not only that, but personal exploration that may have veered far off the beaten track, visited exotic locations, and poured all waters back into the vessel of their own embodied work. They are curious. They are eclectic. They have lived their yoga and witnessed its metamorphosis through different phases of life, so they know that a really serviceable practice is adaptable and unfixed from any particular mooring. For this teacher, what the body discloses is always trusted information. Somatic reflection has long ago overflowed the discreet space of daily practice time and become a way of being, and a key point of reference for action. Out of this lively and pragmatic personal practice proceeds their teaching practice, which therefore has a depth, an authenticity, and a clear and reliable integrity. This teacher knows that kindness and the capacity to listen are what really matter, and that this simple human relatedness is the beginning and the end of teaching yoga.

The total hours worked of a teacher who has taught intensively for two years may be the same as that of a part-time teacher of 10 years' duration, but the 10-year teacher has had time to live into their teaching, to develop, reflect, metabolise, experiment and refine. The slow beat of year rolling over year is important. The 10-year teacher is seasoned, and this makes a difference.

Ten years seems to be a significant landmark in many teaching lives. One of my own teachers told me that in interviewing movement professionals who had been working in their field for several decades, it emerged that all had undergone a significant shift in their orientation to teaching around the 10-year mark. This chimes with my own experience, and when I asked some long-time yoga teachers, many (but not all) agreed. They talked about feeling more at home, creative, self-directed and intuitive in their second decade of teaching, and one (Amanda Coulson) described 'letting the muse of yoga into my classes'.

For this reason, I've chosen to gear this chapter towards teachers with at least a decade's worth of teaching under their belt. That's not to say that none of it will resonate with you if you're a newer teacher, but I'm pretty sure if you come back when you've completed your first decade, you will read it differently, and you will have a fresh set of responses.

Phases of life: the four *ashramas*

Everything gives way and nothing stays.

Heraclitus

One challenge of being a long-term yoga teacher is remaining supple and alive to the shifts that need to happen as we travel through the different phases of life. In the traditional Hindu view, these are formulated as four phases: student (*brahmacharya*), householder (*grihasta*), retired person (*vanaprasthya*) and renunciate (*samnyasa*). Most often, the *ashramas* are not discrete stages but overlap and cross-fade into each other, so that as experienced teachers we might be continuing to build training and workshop programmes while also beginning to drop less specialist work and find more spaces for rest, quiet time and pursuing personal interests; or we may be mostly retired but continuing to teach a couple of long-standing classes and invest energy in our local yoga community.

Stepping back and handing on

A lot of life goes into laying professional foundations and evolving a praxis as a yoga teacher, then developing, refining and substantiating what we have established. It can be difficult and painful to detach identity from profession, to make space and let things go, but there are also opportunities for joy and freedom here. If you believe the internet, yoga teachers are an immortal and ageless breed. When I Googled 'yoga teacher retirement', the top hits were all articles on 'the oldest yoga teacher in the world'. These amazing women (they were all women) are still teaching in their nineties and one-hundreds. Truly an inspiration if you want to go on working indefinitely. But it strikes me that there's a sickness in a culture so loud and enthusiastic about a version of age that closely resembles youth. I'm looking forward to the natural process of slowing down, releasing responsibility, and turning towards a more contemplative way of life.

The internet is chocker with advice on how to become a yoga teacher, but pretty short on suggestions for how to retire, especially if you've always had a low income, as many yoga teachers do. Jessica Garbett has a very useful fact sheet on pensions and retirement at Yoga Tax.[1] I'm no financial expert and I'm not quite yet at the point of dissolving the mandala I've drawn in the sand. However, I have managed to stay solvent – just – for 56 years, through illness, disability and bringing up a child, mainly thanks to a combination of sheer determination and ingenuity, with a sprinkling of pure good luck. So I'm choosing to trust. Our best resources are sometimes not material.

Into the forest

The *ashrama* of renunciate (*samnyasa*) calls us to unhitch entirely from social ties and possessions, slip free of all identities and live as a wandering mendicant or in the forest. Nowadays, it may be a forest of metaphor, but in some way all of us will undergo the process of dismantling and dispersing that precedes the final unknotting of our physical body. If we have practised the yoga that features in magazines and on social media, centred on eternal gains in health and physical capacity, the forest may be a dark, strange and terrifying place. But if we have been engaged over decades in a moving exploration of many landscapes of being, my guess is that we may feel more comfortable here, more blessed and ready to let go.

REFLECTION

- Where do you place yourself in the map of the four *ashramas*? What have you moved through? What are you moving towards? Are you still in the building phase or are you already starting to dissolve and disperse some of what you have created? How has this process been for you so far?

- Have you made any preparations – financial, practical, emotional or spiritual – for retirement? Are there preparations you would like to make?

- What do you look forward to in the present or coming *ashrama*? Is there anything you are afraid of?

Advantages of an ageing body

I am 62 years old. I started yoga when I was 19 and have been teaching for 27 years. About nine years ago, not long after my mum died, I woke up one morning with an urge to go out and dig, which I did. It was a revelation. It was my yoga, my meditation, my practice. Now, if I'm completely honest, if I had to choose between an asana *practice and a stint in the garden, I'd opt for the garden. It's incredibly hard work, but it settles the fluctuations of my mind, which, as Patanjali suggests, is the true purpose of yoga.*

Ellen Lee[2]

There is most often a breadth, spaciousness and ease in an elder yoga practice. It can encompass physical challenge and take pleasure in the body's continuing capacities, but it usually isn't grasping after gymnastic feats. Senior ashtanga vinyasa teacher Richard Freeman, who has been a student of yoga since 1968 and done an acrobatic *asana* or two in his time, describes his present practice with characteristic humour:

I chant a little bit most every day. I enjoy going through the meaning of the chant, but mostly I like the music of it, humming away and making nice melodies. It places all the other practices in context. I also do some *pranayama* and sitting meditation every day. Of course, as I've grown older and dealt with injuries, some of which came from yoga, others which are just due to life, I have modified my [physical] practice. I still practise *asana* every day. I would say it resembles the classical series which Pattabhi Jois taught, but it's segments of the series. If I could, I would definitely go through all seven series [laughs], but there's not enough time in the day![3]

Where practice is sincere and authentic, any sense of loss is mitigated by the knowledge that what makes way gives space for subtler, richer, deeper experiences of moving. When we have practised in a spirit of ongoing enquiry, we are able to carry that same enlivening curiosity over into exploration of the process of ageing and practising itself. David Garrigues, another ashtanga vinyasa teacher of many years says:

I am choosing to approach my studies as though there is particular value in allowing my practice to be a mirror that reflects to me the process of going from youth to elder.[4]

That's not to say that the process of ageing with *asana* is pain-free or straightforward. The pleasure and relative serenity of mature practice is often hard-won. We may be called to re-evaluate both *sadhana* and *svadharma* at a fundamental level, revisit our core intentions and make difficult changes. As our physical practice gradually comes adrift from that of our younger students, there may be all sorts of emotions to negotiate. At one and the same time we may experience nostalgia, jealousy and relief that we no longer feel the need to practise gymnastic postures in long stints.

As their personal practice metamorphoses, some teachers choose to shift their teaching along with it. Derek (age 62) says:

> I've always taught a strong, challenging form of yoga, but I'm no longer able to practise like this, and I find I'm also naturally gravitating towards teaching slower, gentler classes.

Other teachers continue to offer the full range of physical practices to the full range of people, irrespective of whether they still practise them or not. I started out in the ballet world, where it is understood that senior teachers and coaches are no longer able to do a professional class or dance complex and challenging steps, but that over their professional life they have accrued a wealth of experience that is invaluable to performing dancers. I tend to feel this way in the Mysore room. It doesn't matter whether I still…it matters that I have engaged daily with these movements over many years.

It also matters that the Mysore room has available an elder teacher who is engaged in finding pathways for being in meaningful practice. Very often, Mysore teachers don't know (because they haven't been there and haven't had it modelled for them) how to go on teaching older practitioners in a way that continues to offer them rich and interesting routes to pursue, rather than always and only subtracting from their physical practice. Some practitioners choose to leave the ashtanga system, but others drift away because they no longer receive much in the Mysore room, and there is a sense that it's a place for younger and more gymnastic bodies. Unfortunately, this loss of one half of the practising population tips the centre of the room way off balance.

We live in a culture obsessed with looking, staying and feeling young, and in denial about the realities of ageing and death. Perhaps nowhere is this more evident than in the media profile of yoga: all those buff, youthful bodies becoming ever buffer and apparently more youthful. There is an implicit belief that if we can just stay fit enough, we can outrun physical decline. Partly due to the strange trajectory and demographic of popular yoga, which makes it very heavy on 20- or 30-something teachers, there is a dearth of elder teachers modelling genuine physical practice into older life. Not advertorial *faux* older life, with fashionably tinted grey hair and a 'maintained' physique, but older life that is a touch incontinent if it sneezes, and has to do some mobilisation before jumping out of bed in the morning. (That's me.)

I think we have to understand that our current view of yoga is thoroughly lopsided. Yoga is not about constant increase in wellness, fitness, flexibility and general physical capacity; it's about a whole-life journey. This encompasses gaining physical prowess and it also encompasses losing it. The losing phase is just as much yoga as the gaining one. A teacher whose only experience of a complex posture is mastering it has only received one half of the teaching that posture has to offer; the other half is in the long, slow and complex process of letting it go. Our students need opportunities to receive the fullness of this teaching: not only those who are themselves in the second half of life, but also those who are currently young and athletic. The freight of it gives depth and grounding to what otherwise becomes an elite fitness programme.

Physical limitation

Being a yoga practitioner in a hypermobile body, I've found the alterations of ageing less of a jolt than I think I might have done with normal collagen. I've always been going round in circles and making 'progress' in an interesting and complex sort of way, with constant pitstops for mending and recalibration. While I used to be frustrated by the many halts and hitches that characterise physical activity for the hypermobile (no such thing as linear progress here), I grew to love working with limitation. It impels me to let go of preconceived objectives and get creative, to explore new things and find different ways of staying in movement. With shifts in our abilities comes enquiry into how our movement practice may need to change. As artist Robert Rauschenberg says:

> When you work with what's available, the restrictions aren't limitations, they're just what you happen to be working with.

With shifts in our abilities comes enquiry. How are we moving? Why are we moving? What is beneficial now? Longevity as a mover entails the kind of determination that is shot through with intelligence, a mind that is dextrous and flexible and willing to play. The transforming grace is in the capacity to find delight in all of this, because, really, it's much more fun than marching to the beat of somebody else's choreography.

REFLECTION

- How has your body changed over the years? Has your practice had to shift to accommodate these changes? Has this been reflected in your teaching? If so, how?

- How do you envisage your physical practice developing in coming decades? Do you envisage that your teaching will change too? How do you think this might look?

- What advantages, if any, has ageing brought to your teaching? What do you have to offer now that you didn't as a younger teacher? What difficulties, if any, has ageing entailed?

Despairing of the current yoga scene

The countless stories of enthusiastic students loving their first-ever class and immediately running off to do the cheapest, most conveniently located 200-hour training, and within seconds of that jumping in with their superb business plan, leading retreats, corporate classes, one-to-ones, yoga therapy... I've found myself feeling less and less inclined to engage with the wider yoga world, sticking to occasional studies and connection with only those teachers who genuinely seem to still be quietly beavering away, some on the sidelines, some on the international circuit, who are still sharing inspiringly and from a place of real depth and integrity.

Jane Sleven (yoga teacher)

Jane Sleven started teaching in 1981, which was also the year I did my first yoga class. In 1981, yoga happened almost exclusively in community spaces. There weren't any yoga studios, and gyms were for boxing and bodybuilding. Yoga was deeply untrendy. Leggings hadn't been invented, and 'yoga wear' was a concept in some dim and distant dystopian future. Should you have a designed-for-the-purpose yoga mat, the colour choices were either pale turquoise or...pale turquoise. Otherwise, you had an off-cut of carpet underlay.

The yoga 'scene' has changed beyond all recognition in 39 years, and at an escalating speed over the last 10 or 15, as yoga has become subsumed inexorably into the new mega-bucks fitness and wellness industries. The range of yoga products on offer is mindblowing. Not only are there unnumberable brands and varieties of mat (the best-performing of which in 2018, according to reviews.com, come in at between £80 and £125),[5] there are also bags, towels, blankets, jewellery, organic mat cleaners… (Let me tell you a secret, you can put it in the washing machine.) Then there are the 'teachers' who barely have any practice experience and the programmes that profess to train them. And social media… Don't even get me started.

If you see yoga as the stretching component of your fitness programme, it's all good here. But if yoga is for you a set of ethical propositions and a means of living in a more rigorously examined and sustainable way, if it is a body-based tool for reconnecting with what is essentially meaningful to us as human beings…then it's hard not to despair of all the self-promoting fluff and rampant commodification. When one chain yoga retailer offers a class called 'Gin Yin', combining 'two of the great ways to relax, yin yoga and high quality gin',[6] you might be forgiven for feeling it must be the end of days.

So what, in the midst of all this, of the teacher of serious intent? Jane Sleven says:

> As for me, I genuinely don't know whether I still need to be out there, sharing my own current approach to yoga, movement, and wellness of body and mind. No goats, no beer, no business plan, just a place to move and breathe with awareness and cultivate self-awareness that will spread its warmth and good will first inwards, then outwards to the world.

Sometimes it does indeed feel tempting to retire gracefully, leaving the field to those more commercially aggressive contenders.

Some teachers feel that there will always be a student group for know-ledgeable, experienced teachers, grounded in practice and committed to offering their students a teaching of substance. I used to feel this way myself, but now I'm not so sure. Over recent years, my own classes have become increasingly financially unviable. One issue is point of entry. The vast majority of new students get gobbled up by the large, commercial yoga and fitness concerns, because these are highly visible and because they offer huge economies of scale. While a small number of these dabbling yogis will get hooked and move on to other yoga settings where they can access subtler teachings, my experience is that they are few. The norm nowadays actually seems to be to go from initial engagement at a gym or chain studio to teacher training within a couple of years. It's a nought to 100 culture, which bypasses the body of experience lying in the middle ground, and misses important relationships with regular, long-term teachers.

The knock-on here is the further saturation of the market with independent yoga classes, some excellent and others of dubious value, which further exacerbates the problem of visibility. Teachers of Jane's generation will remember advertising in corner shops and local print magazines (and sticking on stamps and addressing envelopes to let students know about class dates and workshops). When I started teaching, relatively recently, in 2003, yoga teachers were just beginning to acquire websites. Given that there were relatively few of us, even in urban areas, just having a website was sufficient to be found by potential students. Word of mouth worked well, because people with an interest in yoga knew about all the classes locally, and often had a good idea of who taught what, and where there were specialisms. There wasn't much competition between yoga teachers – at least, not in my area – because there was no need for it. Obviously, this situation has drastically changed.

My experience, I think, has also been significantly coloured by autism. When I first set out, the professional life of an independent yoga teacher was pretty autism-friendly. There was a lot of room for running the business in unusual and creative ways, and many approaches worked, including eccentric ones. You didn't have to be especially on the ball with marketing, and you could pretty much focus on the actual job. I notice that those independent teachers who are making a reasonable income these days are often those with the will and the capacity to collaborate successfully, for example, with online teaching platforms, with workplace HR (human resources) managers wanting corporate yoga, or with the major studios (particularly valuable in that they offer a degree of platforming from which to launch other ventures). But collaboration is tricky for autistic teachers. There are misunderstandings. Those managing retreat centres, gyms, studios, and so on often lack the capacity to interpret autistic communication – and vice versa. Autistic people are often not able to meet ordinarily accepted demands, which for us are overwhelming and lead, cumulatively and over time, to burn-out.

Social media grind

Once upon a time, the job of a yoga teacher was…teaching yoga. It was pretty simple. Teachers taught, by and large, because they were enthralled by the process of somatic exploration, challenged and engaged by yoga philosophies, and inspired to pass on to others these tools for embodied growth and awareness. Yoga was not a career, and it carried no kudos, so choosing to teach it was almost perverse. Yoga culture was supremely unconcerned with image, and while there were print listings for classes and workshops, there was no avenue for rampant self-promotion. Nowadays, the rampant self-promotion is obligatory, and the pressure to position oneself as a product and maintain online presence has become the blacking factory of yoga teaching in the gig economy. In her *New York Times* article 'Everything is for sale now. Even us', writer Ruth Whippman describes experiences that will be familiar to many yoga teachers:

> Like many modern workers, I find that only a small percentage of my job is now actually doing my job. The rest is performing a million acts of unpaid micro-labour that can easily add up to a full-time job in itself. Tweeting and sharing and schmoozing and blogging. Liking and commenting on others' tweets and shares and schmoozes and blogs. Ambivalently 'maintaining a presence on social media', attempting to sell a semi-fictional, much more appealing version of myself in the vain hope that this might somehow help me sell some actual stuff at some unspecified future time.[7]

According to Karen Mozes, co-leader of *Yoga Journal*'s online Business of Yoga course:

> Your personal journey behind why [sic] you started your career is the most authentic part of you… Once you have crafted your signature story, that should be the foundation of your message in everything you do.[8]

In the view of yoga teacher and podcaster J. Brown, 'Right now, authenticity sells better than anything'.[9] Back in the day, the way a teacher taught just was authentic, because it was the way they taught. Nowadays, in a paramount irony, authenticity is itself fictionalised. Sanitised, emptied of meaning and moral complexity, tanned and toned, it is repurposed as a sales pitch.

If I sound pessimistic, it's because I am, for the short term anyway. As long as yoga is trending, it's going to be puffed up with hot air. But fashion is fickle, and cultural inflation inevitably collapses in on itself in the end. Perhaps, eventually, when the bottom has fallen out of the health and fitness market, and those interested in yoga only for its commmodity value or coolness quotient have moved on, we will be able to return to a quieter and more balanced approach to yoga practice. I hope so.

REFLECTION

■ How do you relate to the current yoga scene? Are you a part of it? At a tangent? Largely outside? Has this changed over the years?

- How has the changing social role and positioning of yoga affected you as a teacher? Has it been largely beneficial, destructive or neutral? How do you see this evolving in the future?

- What is your relationship with social media? Do you use it? Ignore it? How has social media helped/hindered you in your work as a teacher?

The death of your teacher

My long-term teacher died a couple of years ago, and as I've got older the pool of those with more experience than me has become smaller and smaller. How do I find a new teacher? Or is it time to become teacher-less? Can I really be my own support?

Eileen

It can be a surprise to look for senior teachers for guidance and realise that they are all your peers. The reality of elderhood is often very different from the all-pervading wisdom we imagined as a green new yogi, and hard to recognise. When a loved and long-term teacher dies, our grief may be compounded by the loss of the role of student-devotee. We may feel rudderless and flounder. At the same time, there may be a heady sense of freedom and the beginnings of expansion into self-authority.

Finding your internal teacher

Be a lamp unto yourself.

The Buddha, traditional last words

I've always been my favourite teacher, and I've always had to test received teachings against the litmus of my own experience. Autistic people are (mostly) natural autodidacts: focused, self-sufficient and happy to get on with things alone. I taught myself Russian when I was 16, and I have taught myself Sanskrit. When I can follow my own thread, mark out for myself the territory and press into my own exploration, I feel liberated, as if there is finally enough room to stretch and to breathe.

I've received valuable information, support, encouragement and all the good relational stuff from a variety of wonderful teachers, but I've often felt like an anchorite in a leaky coracle. Because it is just this, to practise:

the voyage, the vast expanse of the sea, the unpredicatability of the waves, the leaks in the vessel. All of this is important. It's through this paddling out every day, for years and years, that we become teachers with something to offer our students beyond an architecture of postures, which is not in itself yoga, but simply a context and an invitation for yoga to occur.

If you have practised regularly and sincerely in this way, the teacher you need is already folded into you and waiting to unfurl. This teacher does not look like the one you have lost; it looks like you. It teaches like you; it moves in your shapes and uses your vocabulary. In the space vacated is an opportunity for re-evaluation, change and growth. This is the natural cell division necessary for a lineage, school or organisation to renew and proliferate in a healthy way.

It's often the death of a teacher that compels the transition into maturity for the student. In all long-term teacher–student relationships there comes a point where it's no longer possible to sustain in honesty relationships of inequality with our teachers, because the differential in knowledge, skills and experience that was there when we were a new practitioner no longer exists. At this point, if your teacher is flexible and democratic, they may welcome you as a colleague. If they are not willing to see and acknowledge the shift that has occurred, maturation for the student may entail a painful and distressing rift. I've witnessed this several times in organisations with a determinedly top-down structure. On the plus side, these splits have disseminated many fertile seeds, resulting in some creative new forms and practice structures. The emotional cost of separation has often been high, though.

Peer network as teacher

Thich Nhat Hanh has famously said that the next Buddha will be the *sangha*. As I've got older, relationship with peers has become increasingly important to me as a source of support, collaboration and testing of ideas. Some of my significant peers teach yoga, many of them are elders in allied professions, but we all share an orientation to our work and a set of attitudes about what it means to be offering embodied practice in a way that honours the student/client and their own capacity for emergence.

The brilliant thing about peer support is that, like water, it naturally and spontaneously overflows the boundary with friendship, washing all waters into one jar. Because all life is in the jar, the potential for creativity is large. The other brilliant thing is that peers, by definition, have parity. They are therefore likely to ask questions and call one another out. The normal checks and balances of normal relationships, happening within a wider community, are in operation. Those sociopathic teachers with their programmes of various kinds of abuse have generally separated themselves off at an early stage from ordinary community and have therefore been exempt from the rough and tumble of comment and assessment that happens in well-functioning groups of equals and, in the best-case scenario, acts to quash megalomaniac tendencies.

REFLECTION

- Have you ever experienced the death of an important teacher? How was this for you emotionally? What was the impact on you as a teacher? How did you move forwards?

- Do you tend to look upwards towards a teacher or sideways towards peers and community? How does this orientation serve you? Are there ways in which it does not serve you?

When your teacher is outed as abusive

I think...it is important to remember that we all live in glass houses. By that, I mean we all commit acts that in retrospect we might regret: certainly this is true for me. I have definitely done actions that I might describe in terms of regret – that I wish I hadn't done.

Norman Blair[10]

The list of high-profile teachers exposed for serious misdemeanours is now long, and many of us will have been in some sort of relationship, however loose, with an abusive teacher or lineage. In 2018, Pattabhi Jois, the progenitor of my own main practice, ashtanga vinyasa, was outed as sexually abusive, financially dishonest and injurious in his use of physical adjustments.[11] For those practitioners who were in a close and ongoing relationship with Jois, whose professional status rests upon having been Certified or Authorised by the former Shri K. Pattabhi Jois Ashtanga Yoga Institute (KPJAYI), who may have witnessed sexual abuse and smoothed away the evidence in their own minds, there has been a huge amount of cognitive dissonance, resulting for some in ongoing denial and for others in positive re-evaluation and re-orientation.

My own relationship with Pattabhi Jois and what was known as KPJAYI is a bit more ambivalent. I'm not a Certified or Authorised teacher, and beyond that pale I've been doing things progressively more and more creatively over the years. I've never been to Mysore (where KPJAYI was located), and neither have any of my long-term teachers. I met Pattabhi Jois twice, at classes on his regular London tours. On the whole, I found these events more like a circus than a practice space, and never attended regularly. I had no intimation of any sexual abuse. Perhaps if I were allistic, I might have heard in-talk or read between the lines. The dangerousness of the adjustments, particularly for hypermobile people like me and many of my students, was evident to me from the get-go, and risk of injury was a major reason why I never went to Mysore, and advised hypermobile students against it too. I guess I also knew that I can't help bringing a certain amount of dissidence to the party. I was pretty sure that KPJAYI was not elastic enough to be able to include that, in the way that some more supple organisations can.

For the many teachers working at grass-roots level, the crimes of gurus and often super-star teachers will feel remote and of little relevance to their own classes and teachings. While I can't speak to the experience of those teachers who have been devout disciples, or who are victims/survivors of guru abuse, I can offer some suggestions for those common-or-garden teachers who have always done their best to uphold ethical standards but who have discovered that those in the upper echelons of the practice lineage did not.

- Be alert for abusive attitudes, behaviours or approaches that may have been refracted into your own teaching. These may be subtle assumptions or ways of doing things that fail to respect the student and erode healthy relational norms. They may have been transparent and become visible only as the old order crumbles and everyone's filters change. For example, it was usual in Mysore to give strong physical adjustments without enquiring about possible contraindications or asking for feedback from students. There was an implicit belief that 'teacher knows best'. Consequently there has been a tendency throughout ashtanga teaching to adjust overly hard, irrespective of body type and without regard for consent. Teachers in the ashtanga system need to make space for talking to each student, finding out about them as a whole person, and ensuring that we work in collaboration with them so that all our physical interactions are as sensitive as possible.

- Look to what is essentially good and valuable in the practices. Focus on how you can develop this, while stripping away what were aspects of abusive power, or just ill-informed and unhelpful.

- Be clear and honest with students who ask questions about abuses within the organisation, school or lineage, and share reliable sources of information. How much it's appropriate to address senior teachers' behaviour in our own general classes is a judgement call. If I mentioned Pattabhi Jois to many of my students, they wouldn't know who I was talking about, so banging on to them about what went down in Mysore feels gratuitous. Consider sharing relevant articles on your professional social media, and be open to discussing them with students who are interested or concerned.

- Back in the day, teachers believed (and I was one of them) that an ashtanga vinyasa practice was perfectly balanced and provided all anyone might need on physical, ethical and philosophical levels. Seen in the clear light of day, it's clear that it isn't and it doesn't. Nor does any form of yoga. Be honest about what students may need in order to balance their practice, and point them towards resources. Encourage students to experiment with Pilates, core fitness work and strength training, and to read widely across many different fields. Emotional intelligence and neurology come to mind as especially important, but there's lots of relevant material out there.

- Encourage students to practise *viveka*, discrimination. Positive teaching experiences are collaborative and facilitate the student in making their own experiential exploration; they do not require the student to give themselves over wholly to the teacher or to introject the teacher's received word.

- Look to create community through peers (see above, 'Finding your internal teacher', and 'Peer network as teacher') and within the spaces that you yourself hold (see below, 'Creating practice communities').

- Consider seeking regular professional mentorship/supervision, one-to-one, with an experienced teacher or other appropriate person. This can be invaluable in opening your eyes to blind spots, as well as offering encouragement and support.

REFLECTION

▦ Have you been in relationship with an abusive teacher, lineage or organisation? How has this affected you as a practitioner? And as a teacher?

▦ How do you encourage students to be discerning in their relationships with teachers and discriminating in the teachings they choose to take on? Are there other things you would like to try?

Creating practice communities

The community I've built goes beyond the mat. Many of us have become great friends. I buy my eggs from one student, have my hair done by another (half the class now seems to get their hair done by her). People make cakes, pottery and bath salts for each other, and one of the guys is everybody's taxi driver. I've visited students in hospital and even put some of them up for a few days.

Shena Grigor (MadDogYoga)[12]

As I've mentioned elsewhere in this book (see Chapter 4, 'Classes or communities'), my passion as a teacher is for creating practice spaces that are more than classrooms where students come to learn the skills and tools of embodiment, but are also communities where members forge real and sustaining relationships with each other that extend out into their whole lives. Because such relationships are founded in embodied presence, facilitated and modelled by the teacher, they have the potential to be capacious containers, able to hold difficult human experiences – grief, illness, relationship transitions and so on – in a spirit of witness and companionship. Where family and social support networks are unable to bear the pain or discomfort of a situation, and may try to shut it down by imposing advice or talking over the person in distress, the quiet listening of body-centred community can be a mainstay and a huge relief.

With a few particular exceptions, I find the current standard template for a yoga class poorly designed for meaningful teaching. This is why I teach mostly Mysore-style. I want to be able to have an individual relationship with students. I want to be able to give different practices to different people, and I want to be able to include people with widely differing physical capacities in a way that serves each of them equally and uniquely. While everyone is travelling solo, in my Mysore room I also promote an ethos of collaboration and comradeship. Each mat may be a single-occupation island, but it's also part of an archipelago. There are plenty of informal opportunities for students to teach me and to teach each other, by discussing what works for them in particular postures, sharing practice tips, and pooling experiences. I love this democratisation of the space where yoga happens, and I've learnt a lot from my students.

I think that community is an important antidote to the rampant colonisation of yoga by big corporations and to the orgiastic self-promotion of #yoga. I'm not talking about community as represented in yoga advertorial here, with its spew of airbrushed images of cute disabled children and coffee-coloured black people. No, I'm talking about the community that happens when we do our damnedest to actually include people who, for whatever reason, are hard to reach out to and challenging to integrate. This means we have to keep opening our ears to listen when most of our fibres are straining not to hear. It means we have to let go of some of our cherished assumptions about how things are supposed to be in a yoga class. While community of this kind isn't wholly outside the standard monetary system, other forms of exchange are also possible here. Relationship is prioritised, and values such as love, affection and mutual respect trump unfeasibly large financial gain.

REFLECTION

- Are you part of a practice-related community? What do you offer to the community and what do you receive?

- Do you foster community in your teaching? If so, how do you do this? What benefits do you feel that community offers to your students? And to you?

Burn-out

'Oh, you're a yoga teacher! That must be so relaxing!' Ever heard that? Yes, I thought so. The reality, of course, is somewhat different. Burn-out can be mostly about our physical capacity to get up every morning, maintain a full schedule, and fulfil our responsibilities to work, family, and so on. It's a kind of 'the spirit is willing but the flesh is weak' scenario. I have three fatiguing genetic conditions and have experienced serious burn-out of this kind, after which I was ill for a long time. For most of my adult life I've felt as if I'm trying to balance an equation that is fundamentally out of kilter. I never have quite enough energy to make a basic living and feel fully rested and ready to go. Then there's the burn-out that's more like reluctance or resistance. You're just fed up to the back teeth with yoga. You don't want to do yoga, teach yoga, see yoga, or hear anything at all about yoga. Senior Iyengar yoga teacher Theresa Elliott describes this experience:

> For some odd reason, I feel like I have a repetitive stress injury in my brain from constantly thinking about yoga. At age 54, I am showing clear signs of a burn-out. There are topics I can no longer bear. Please, do not bring up vegetarianism, 'opening' the heart, fasting to get rid of toxins, or casually bandy about the word 'spiritual' within earshot unless you have at least three possible working definitions of the word, one of which you actually believe.[13]

Burn-out can feel overwhelming, but one thing I've learnt about it is that making small changes can create significant shifts. These are a few things that have helped me, and some other teachers, in times of exhaustion:

- Your daily practice time is sacred space for you. Don't allow work to encroach on it – ever.

- Your practice is your resource. If you're exhausted, make it restful and replenishing – blankets, bolsters and supported restorative postures. If you feel reluctant to get on your mat, you probably need to change what you do in your practice time. Never use your practice time to prepare for classes. This is not work time; it's time for you. (For more on this, see Chapter 2, 'Maintaining your own practice'.)

- Yoga nidra, yoga nidra, yoga nidra. Listening to a recorded nidra as you go to sleep at night offers an opportunity for deep rest, and can be helpful with insomnia.

- Take a week off – completely off. Yes, you can. When I used to teach in the evening, I scheduled classes in six-week blocks and left a week empty in between each one. This was my half-term. Sometimes I did some daytime work during it, but if I needed a week completely off, one was always available at regular intervals.

- Sometimes the problem isn't the number of hours worked, but the way our work fits together – or doesn't. Look at your schedule and consider how you may be able to make more sense out of it geographically or in terms of when you choose to teach (only during the day or only in the evenings, for example). Be prepared to eliminate work that doesn't fit or isn't worth the effort. Even if you can't make all the changes you want immediately, working towards them will give you a sense of relief and progressive improvement. Although this kind of refinement is most often something we do earlier on in our working life, it can be useful to revisit it periodically. As an experienced teacher we can end up with work we continue to do because we've done it forever, even though it no longer really serves us.

- Take stock of where your output in energy is out of whack with the income you gain in return. This may mean offering fewer group classes and more trainings or therapeutic sessions or whatever is your specialism.

- Be aware of where you may be giving your services away un-intentionally. This can create a surprisingly large energy drain. For more information, see below, 'Dealing with requests for free advice'.

- Know that you are not responsible for everyone and everything, even if it feels as if you are. No one is indispensable. Sometimes we need to step out and allow a client to feel themselves adrift or a group to crumble so that one cycle can come to an end and a new thing can emerge.

- If you don't have time to eat properly and look after your basic needs, you're working too much. This is foundational and more important than anything else. If you don't create more space in your day, you will get ill.

- Make sure you have at least two consecutive days completely off every week. Yes, you do need this, even if your working days aren't nine-to-five. The days need to be consecutive so that you have time to switch off completely from work. Think about it: everyone else has a weekend.

- Know that you do have time to prioritise your own well-being and that doing so is essential if you don't want to become much more seriously ill and incapacitated in the future. As Judith Lasater says, 'If you don't have time for *savasana*…you really need to practise *savasana*.'

- Theresa Elliott exchanged teaching yoga for a job in a mall. If you're fed up with yoga, have a break. Go and do something completely different – and go with a big-sky mind. Perhaps you will return to your life as a yoga teacher, or maybe this will be a permanent new trajectory. Anything could happen.

Elder yoga teacher Jude Murray has an excellent free eBook on preventing and coping with burn-out called, *Don't Be a Leaky Bucket – Anti-Burn-out Workbook.*[14]

REFLECTION

▪ Have you ever experienced burn-out? What factors – emotional, situational, practical – contributed? How did you recover?

▪ Do you currently feel depleted and close to burn-out? What might you need to restore your energy? How might you be able to receive some of this? Think wide open and creatively.

Dealing with requests for free advice

I've taught yoga to children with learning difficulties for many years, and I've become quite well-known in this area of work. The problem is, I'm inundated with emails from parents and teachers who I've never met asking for advice. They don't seem to realise that they're asking for specialist help that it takes me time and energy to provide.

Jayne

If every person who ever contacted me requesting advice about hypermobility had actually been a paying client, I would have waved goodbye to the mortgage and receded contentedly into a life of leisure some while ago. For a long time, I was the only person (that I knew of) working with yoga and hypermobility. Hypermobile people are often in a lot of pain, suffering from multiple syndromes and desperate to find someone who can help them to move in a way that may initiate improvement rather than make things worse. They are also sometimes very comprehensive in their elaborations of the difficulties they want me to address.

There's a general assumption in our culture that yoga teachers are a font of all-giving charity. It's an assumption that yoga teachers ourselves often share. Many of us feel duty-bound to help anyone who comes to us in need, and may go out of our way to do so, without asking for anything in return.

Obviously, this is neither personally sustainable nor conducive to running a successful business.

The following are a few simple guidelines for deciding what you can feasibly offer and to whom. These are geared to approaches received by email or messaging. For suggestions about how to manage student requests for advice before and after classes, see Chapter 4, 'Setting boundaries around student time'.

Do you wanna?

If your immediate response to a request is one of dread, overwhelm or depression...you know what to do! Follow your instinct here. Some requests, however, pique curiosity, involve some kind of *quid pro quo*, or can be quickly and easily met. I'm always more likely to offer help if the person has limited themselves to one or two specific questions, if they have expressed respect for the time involved in responding, and if they have acknowledged a boundary around what I can offer for free.

Can you ethically?

In many instances, it's not possible to address issues raised without working individually with the person. It goes without saying that a doctor, physiotherapist or other medical professional would never diagnose or offer prognoses without having met the patient. Nor can a yoga teacher evaluate a person's movement patterns in this way or (assuming appropriate training) offer emotional work.

Define the parameters

It's important to be clear about what you are and are not willing to offer for free and how you are willing to offer it. For example, in certain circumstances I'm willing to email a few general pointers for hypermobile yoga practitioners and directions to some references. I'm not willing to call anyone or be called by them. (Be aware of the propensity for a phone call to turn into a free consultation.) Unless this is a connection I'm genuinely interested in pursuing, I'm also not willing to meet up for coffee. I'm often asked if I can recommend a hypermobility-friendly teacher in...Milwaukee...Honolulu...Wellington...Milan...or somewhere else I haven't been and don't know a soul. My response is:

I'm sorry, but I don't currently run certificated training programmes for teachers, so I can't recommend anyone. Look for an experienced teacher with a sound biomechanical sense who has a good reputation in your area and who offers a lot of individual attention. Then trust your common sense. Is it helping? If not, look elsewhere. Be aware that it can take many years and lots of attempts to find an appropriate teacher.

Have some basic free resources

I originally wrote 'Hypermobility on the yoga mat'[15] specifically in order to have something to offer hypermobile people who contacted me asking for advice. I naively thought I had it covered. 'Hypermobility on the yoga mat' was widely shared, added to the reading list of a major teacher training, picked up by *Elephant Journal*, and became fairly high-profile. People soon started contacting me because they'd read the article and were after more personalised free advice. When a person has read, watched or listened to your free resources and wants more, this is the moment to direct them towards your paid-for services:

> I'm glad you found the video helpful. You might be interested in the course I'm running…

Respond with grace

If you're feeling particularly pissed off by the amount of requests you've received lately for free help, or by the tone of the one you've just read: *pause!* Don't respond while you're feeling reactive. Your reply needs to be friendly, sympathetic, clear in boundarying what you are (and are not) able to offer, and engaging with regard to your paid-for services:

> Thanks for getting in touch. Each hypermobile person has unique bio-mechanics, so it isn't possible to offer individual advice by email. For general guidelines, have a look at my article 'Hypermobility on the yoga mat'. I also offer occasional hypermobility workshops; you can find details of these at [website address]. Please let me know if you'd like to be added to the workshop email list. If you'd like to book a one-to-one session, I'd be very happy to work with you. Please let me know, and we can arrange a time.

If you're really inundated with questions and queries, make something like this a standard reply email. Cut and paste – you're done.

Journalist Rosie Spinks has a very good article on 'How to politely decline giving advice for free'.[16]

REFLECTION

▣ How do you approach requests for free advice? What predisposes you to offer some help? What predisposes you not to?

▣ Do you need to set better boundaries around how you deal with questions and queries? How might you do this? What kind of support might you need?

Where to now?

For me, essential to being an experienced yoga teacher is feeling comfortable with not knowing, remaining open to change how you teach in line with current findings on movement and anatomy, and being willing to do what others are not to move yoga forwards, away from tradition and towards what honours safety and sacredness.

William George[17]

When I asked experienced teachers what they would like to be included in this chapter, several mentioned the question of where we see ourselves in relation to yoga lineage, history and philosophy, and how we define yoga in a time when the meaning of the word has been exploded.

'Yoga' is indeed a capacious portmanteau, and in this lies both challenge and potential. For me, personally, what defines yoga is a combination of somatic presence, biomechanical intelligence and connection to something bigger than ourselves. Whether or not the practice includes chanting and mantras and New Agey talk is irrelevant to whether it is 'spiritual' or not, because in embodied practice spiritual is immanent. It's immanent in the body, it's immanent in movement, and it's immanent in the field of practice we create when we come together with an intention to move with awareness of all the dimensions of our experience.

Bedizened in narcissistic social media ra-ra and groaning under the weight of commercialism, yoga might seem wrecked, pillaged and desecrated, but it's hard to completely despoil a practice whose deep roots are ancient and shamanic. The green shoots of yoga are protean. Some of the promising new growth is in intelligent engagement with cutting-edge movement research and neuroscience, in trauma work, in community building, in embodied rehabilitation work in prisons, and so on.

Eventually the cash cow's gotta give out, clearing the field for those engaged with somatic explorations of real value. You'd think. You'd hope. Gimme a million 'likes' on that one.

Handing on

I'd like to end this chapter by extending a hand to the new generation. As senior teachers we contribute deep roots and the gravity of experience, but yoga also needs the leven of youth and the effervescence of new possibility – the left field, the unforeseen. To our apprentices and mentees we entrust the future of yoga practice. May you explore widely and teach well.

EXPERIENTIAL WORK: MANY PIECES

I decided to offer collage work for this final piece of experiential work because the form mirrors the exploded nature of where yoga is at now. It also reflects the nature of a long teaching life, which is often less like a single skein and more like a colourful mosaic. This is an exploration you can do purely for pleasure, but you can also use it to learn something about your present relationship with your teaching, with your practice or with the state of yoga as a whole. Thanks to 5Rhythms™ teacher Dilys Morgan Scott for introducing me to this exploration.

You will need:

- Print magazines, leaflets or catalogues - as varied as possible.

- A packet of blank postcards.

- Scissors.

- A stick of glue.

- A clock, watch or timer.

- A quiet space where you won't be interrupted for 30 minutes or so.

1. Prepare by entering the terrain of your body through physical movement - see suggestions for how to do this in Chapter 1.

2. Give yourself 20 minutes. It's important that you don't go over the time limit, because this process is meant to happen at speed - too fast for your thinking mind to be able to do a lot of choosing and evaluating.

3. You are going to use one postcard to make a collage from your print materials. Aim to cover the whole surface of the card. It can be in any style, any colour. Go!

4. When 20 minutes is up, stop. Now look at your collage. What strikes you about it visually? What shapes can you see? Which colours predominate? How does the collage make you feel? Does it reflect anything going on in your life at the moment? Does it offer you any information?

You can make a whole series of collages like this - you will get a whole series of pieces of information. If you make enough collages, you can use them as a pack of divination cards. If you have a problem to resolve or a decision to make, draw a card and see what percolates.

9

Going Forward

Teaching yoga is a life-long journey involving commitment to practice, awareness and investigation into our own unfolding experiences. As senior ashtanga vinyasa teacher Mary Taylor says:

> It is the responsibility of a yoga teacher to keep practising, to keep enquiring both into the subject matter and into themselves, to keep studying and asking questions, and to encourage students to do the same.[1]

This responsibility is a serious one and may come to feel burdensome without the support of teachers, mentors and community. The actual work of teaching yoga, though, can be isolating, offering few routine opportunities to meet with colleagues and mull over professional issues. Lucy says:

> I feel lonely as a yoga teacher. Students look up to me for guidance and encouragement, but I feel that I don't have any support myself. I'm constantly going from gym to studio to gym. I rarely meet any other yoga teachers, never mind have time to make a relationship with them. I'd love to be able to share teaching experiences with someone or ask about problems when they come up now and again.

While it isn't always easy to locate, there is community, connection and mentoring available out there. While some of it costs money to access, there are also ways of receiving support without investing anything financially.

Paid-for mentoring

Most of us feel the need for specialised professional support at certain times in our teaching life. Intrinsic to the role of yoga teacher is the task of holding groups and individuals through all sorts of experiences, some of them challenging. While this is rewarding work, it can be also be exhausting, and if we don't have access to spaces where we are ourselves held, burnout is an inevitability. A growing number of experienced yoga teachers are offering professional mentoring as a paid-for service, both one-to-one and in groups. If you want a regular, structured system of support and can afford to pay for it, this can be a great option.

Be aware that what is available under the mentorship umbrella is quite diverse, so before you commit, check out what your potential mentor is offering and make sure it meets your needs. Ola, one of my one-to-one mentees, told me:

> I've already completed one mentor group. Don't get me wrong, it was good. There was a lot of useful information and skill-building – but it was more like a course. What I really wanted was time to talk about my own difficulties and receive individual feedback. I would have liked to talk more to the other participants and perhaps have had a chance to form more permanent relationships with them, but there wasn't much opportunity for that.

Consider whether your potential mentor has experience with any client groups you specialise in – or would like to: people with mental health issues, children, elders, people wiith cancer, trauma survivors, dancers and performers... Consider, too, which settings your potential mentor has worked in and whether these are a fit for you. If you run your own classes, for example, you may do better with a mentor who has mostly done likewise and has first-hand experience of publicising classes, building a student base, dealing with venues and so on. And a mentor who has focused on working in gyms and studios is going to have valuable experience of the issues that tend to come up in these settings.

Mentoring as supervision

Some mentoring is akin to supervision of the kind a psychotherapist receives. If you work with challenging clients – people with developmental trauma, mental health issues or eating disorders, for example – this type of mentoring is going to be essential, both for your own well-being and for the well-being of your students. Those offering this kind of mentoring are often not only yoga teachers but also yoga therapists, mental health professionals or psychotherapists with specialist training in working with their particular client group. Even if you work only with the general population, this style of mentoring can be very helpful for exploring your relational dynamics with individual students or with particular groups, and for generally understanding a bit more about feelings that arise in the context of teaching and how they play into your attitudes and actions.

Mentoring as training and professional development

This kind of mentor group focuses on filling gaps in skills and offering more advanced training. It usually has a pre-set structure, with modules on, for example, social media marketing, physical adjustments, theming classes, email lists and data protection, writing effective publicity and so on. This type of programme may also offer CEUs (Continuing Education Units).

Mentoring as a space for listening and receiving

The intention of this type of mentor group is to offer teachers the opportunity to speak about their own teaching experiences, in depth and from the heart, within a community of peers. The mentor will mostly listen carefully and ask questions, and may use tools such as mirroring and open-ended questions. The focus is on personal development and enquiry. There may be experiential work (drawing, writing, moving) designed to help the person emerge their own answers. This kind of group is likely to be fluid in content and follow the needs of the students, so no two groups will be the same. There's an emphasis on relationship building and on teaching as a vocation, a practice and an unfolding journey.

Mentoring and support without money exchange

If you can't afford to pay for mentoring, there are still lots of options available.

Informal mentoring by your own yoga teacher

One of the big advantages of receiving mentoring this way is that your own teacher will already have observed your practice over a long period of time and will know you well in this setting. On the downside, while some teachers are extraordinarily generous with their time, it's not realistic to expect the amount of mentoring input from your yoga teacher that you would receive from a paid mentor. It's going to be in-between and around classes, and there will probably not be time for detailed work, extensive skills building, or more subtle exploratory processes.

Apprenticing and assisting

Learning about adjustments and actually doing them are two very different things. As a new teacher, I found the reality of adjusting students really scary. Assisting has helped me learn to adjust according to different body types and to understand that there are no cookie-cutter adjustments.

Mai

If you're a new teacher, apprenticing or assisting can be a great way to receive regular ongoing training and mentoring and have your development as a teacher overseen and helped along by an experienced teacher. A big plus of this situation is that it offers lots of opportunities to practise teaching skills without having to be responsible for looking after a whole class and keep all the plates spinning. Nina, who first apprenticed with me five years ago, and is now my most experienced assistant teacher, says:

Assisting a senior teacher has given me a safe environment to learn and grow during and after my teacher teacher training. I feel very lucky to have had the experience of assisting and learning from different teachers over a period of several years. There's no better way to learn!

I'm mainly an ashtanga vinyasa teacher working in a Mysore setting, where there is a tradition of apprenticeship and where the gains for apprentices and assistant teachers are greater than they may be in the more usual type of yoga class – in which there tends to be a lot less time for the lead teacher to feed back, train and mentor assistants. If you are considering assisting, check out what the class teacher is likely to be able to offer you. As I mentioned in Chapter 2, for some teachers, assisting means taking the money and putting the mats out; for others it may entail teaching some parts of the class under supervision. Before you commit, know what the exchange is and make sure it feels fair to you and that it meets your needs. This will avoid any potential bad feeling in the future. You really don't want to end up at odds with an established teacher in your local area!

In my Mysore programme, an apprentice is usually someone wanting to teach but with no offical training as yet, or a teacher beginning training, or a recently qualified teacher who has no previous practice history with me. Apprentices receive a lot of supervision and are mostly shadowing, observing, asking questions and learning theory, skills and adjustments. An assistant teacher is someone who has practised with me regularly for some time and has either completed a teacher training or done a hefty period of apprenticeship with me, and is gradually becoming more self-sufficient as a teacher in the room. Over time, some of my assistants become very experienced teachers in their own right.

Training and supervising junior teachers does require a considerable amount of extra energy, but I love having them in the Mysore shala. They bring more layers to the compost heap of our practice community – different types of relationship, alternative ways of approach, and different personal styles. All of this diversifies and adds more possibilities to the room. In practical terms, the payback for me becomes greater over time. Mai, another of my assistant teachers, who you heard from at the start of this section, says:

> The Mysore room is a safe environment to keep learning and being inspired, and also to build trust between your peers, your teacher and their students. The sharing of this knowledge is something you cannot find in a classroom or teacher training.

Mentoring, training and feedback is the usual exchange for assisting an experienced teacher – money doesn't generally change hands. In the Mysore programme I run, assistants also receive free classes and the occasional free or reduced-cost workshop. If they are sufficiently experienced, they may also be offered paid class cover and one-to-one students. Apprentices continue to pay for classes. However, there may be situations where it's appropriate for an assistant teacher to receive a monetary payment. Gina, a yoga teacher in one of my mentor groups, had been offered a lucrative corporate gig involving 90 students. There was a lot of complicated getting in and out, name-taking and mat organising that she wanted the assistant to look after, and she knew there wouldn't be much time to offer feedback or training. Although her newly qualified assistant teacher was very willing to help for free, Gina decided to offer her a fee of £30 for her work.

Teacher meet-ups

Many local areas have a regular meet-up event for local teachers. Ask around where you teach or try searching for a Facebook group. If you can't find one, create one yourself. Meet-ups are usually easy-going and relatively simple to organise. Sometimes they are just a get-together in a cafe, or they may involve a free class or mini-workshop donated by one of the member teachers.

Online groups

If you use Facebook, you will find a variety of groups for yoga teachers. Some offer support and mentoring and are nationwide or international, others are more local and offer chances to meet up in real life, to cover and to skills swap.

Final word

While it may initially be difficult to find, there is a lot of support and mentoring available out there. Many elder teachers feel a responsibility to the transmission of yoga of real worth, and are very willing to help junior teachers who show themselves to be genuine, keen to learn and willing to commit.

Good luck with the journey. Remember that there is a true compass in your body. Consult it regularly, and while you may have many unexpected adventures, you will never lose your way.

Further Reading

Bruce Black (2011) *Writing Yoga: A Guide to Keeping a Practice Journal*. Berkeley, CA: Rodmell Press.

Norman Blair (2016) *Brightening Our Inner Skies: Yin and Yoga*. London: MicMac Margins.

T.K.V. Desikachar (1995) *The Heart of Yoga: Developing a Personal Practice*. Rochester, VT: Inner Traditions International.

Donna Farhi (2004) *Bringing Yoga to Life: The Everyday Practice of Enlightened Living*. New York: HarperCollins.

Donna Farhi (2006) *Teaching Yoga: Ethics and the Teacher–Student Relationship*. Berkeley, CA: Rodmell Press.

Jay Fields (2012) *Teaching People Not Poses: 12 Principles for Teaching Yoga with Integrity*. CreateSpace Independent Publishing Platform.

Richard Freeman (2010) *The Mirror of Yoga: Awakening the Intelligence of Body and Mind*. Boston, MA: Shambhala Publications Inc.

Carol Horton and Roseanne Harvey (eds) (2012) *21st Century Yoga: Culture, Politics and Practice*. Chicago, IL: Kleio Books.

B.K.S. Iyengar (2005) *Light on Life: The Journey to Wholeness, Inner Peace and Ultimate Freedom*. Basingstoke and Oxford: Rodale.

Parker Palmer (1997) *The Courage to Teach: Exploring the Inner Landscape of a Teacher's Life*. San Francisco, CA: John Wiley & Sons.

Matthew Remski (2019) *Practice and All Is Coming: Abuse, Cult Dynamics, and Healing in Yoga and Beyond*. Rangiora, New Zealand: Embodied Wisdom Publications.

Matthew Sanford (2006) *Waking: A Memoir of Trauma and Transcendence*. Emmaus, PA: Rodale.

Erich Schiffman (1996) *Yoga: The Spirit and Practice of Moving into Stillness*. New York: Pocket Books, Simon & Schuster.

Mark Singleton (2010) *Yoga Body: The Origins of Modern Posture Practice*. New York: Oxford University Press.

Michael Stone (2008) *The Inner Tradition of Yoga: A Guide to Yoga Philosophy for the Contemporary Practitioner*. Boston, MA: Shambhala Publications Inc.

Kylea Taylor (1995) *The Ethics of Caring: Honouring the Web of Life in Our Professional Healing Relationships*, 2nd edn. Santa Cruz, CA: Hanford Mead Publishers.

About the Author

Jess Glenny is a moving body, teacher, facilitator and therapist based in South East London. She did her first yoga class in 1981 and has been teaching yoga since 2003. She is also a Phoenix Rising yoga therapist and mentors yoga teachers. For more information, see www.embodyyogadance.co.uk

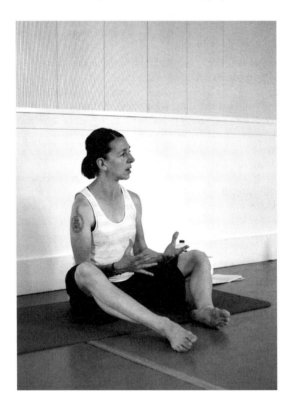

Endnotes

1   Thanks to Theodora Wildcroft for this quotation, which she received from Vedanta teacher Nandana Nagraj.

Introduction

1   For more on the internal locus of ethics, see Chapter 4.

Chapter 1

1   I am grateful to Open Floor teacher Lori Saltzman for creating and sharing the basic material for the 'Phases of becoming' section. Lori developed these ideas from the work of Lillian Katz, a researcher on early education. I have freely adapted this material, so my version is somewhat the same and also different.
2   Bunyan, J. (1678) Pilgrim's Progress.
3   Lizzie Lasater (2018) 'Influence and Evolution.' In Sian O'Neill (ed.) *Yoga Teaching Handbook: A Practical Guide for Yoga Teachers and Trainees*. London and Philadelphia, PA: Singing Dragon.

Chapter 2

1   David Garrigues (no date) 'What I believe makes an effective teacher.' Available at https://davidgarrigues.com/writings/what-i-believe-makes-an-effective-teacher
2   Parker J. Palmer (2017) *The Courage to Teach Guide for Reflection and Renewal*. San Francisco, CA: Jossey Bass.
3   Lizzie Lasater (2018) 'Influence and Evolution.' In Sian O'Neill (ed.) *Yoga Teaching Handbook: A Practical Guide for Yoga Teachers and Trainees*. London and Philadelphia, PA: Singing Dragon.
4   You can find the fact sheets at https://yogatax.co.uk/help
5   See https://yogatax.co.uk/help/general-insurances
6   See www.independentyoganetwork.org
7   www.namaskaram.co.uk/regulation-the-facts
8   Personal communication.
9   For more on the decline in yoga teacher pay, see Norman Blair's important articles 'Let's talk about...' at www.yogawithnorman.co.uk/space/c16a5320fa475530d9583c34fd356ef5/pdfs/lets_talk_about._._._.pdf and 'Let's talk about too...' at www.yogawithnorman.co.uk/space/c16a5320fa475530d9583c34fd356ef5/pdfs/Lets_Talk_About_Too_19_Feb.pdf
10 www.gov.uk/make-money-claim

11 See 'MoreYoga entrepreneurs plan 100 studios for London', www.healthclubmanagement.co.uk/health-club-management-news/More-Yoga-entrepreneurs-plan-100-studios-for-London-/338422

12 https://triyoga.co.uk/discover/work-with-us

13 Most insurers make some stipulations in the general area of duty of care. Litigation against yoga teachers is very rare in the UK, but should a student ever take legal action against you following alleged injury or wrongful advice in your class, you would need to be able to demonstrate that you were attentive to the safety and well-being of the student in your teaching. A completed class joining form, including a student health history, will help to evidence this. (Thanks to Nick Elwell of BGI UK insurers for advice on the insurance- and litigation-related aspects of this section. Any errors are my own.)

Chapter 3

1 Taken from 'The art of verbal communication.' Yoga Journal, 28 August. Available at www.yogajournal.com/teach/the-art-of-verbal-communication

2 Ibid.

3 If you find yourself having to give a lot of technical input in every posture, your class is probably too difficult for your students.

4 A BBC TV children's programme, made in 1971–72.

5 Taken from 'Four tips for ditching yoga speak and finding your voice.' Yoga International. Available at https://yogainternational.com/article/view/4-tips-for-ditching-yoga-speak-and-finding-your-voice

6 Personal communication.

7 '#TimesUp: Ending sexual abuse in the yoga community.' Yoga Journal, 12 February 2018. Available at www.yogajournal.com/lifestyle/timesup-metoo-ending-sexual-abuse-in-the-yoga-community

8 One teacher recently told me they considered touch – any touch – in the yoga room to be 'a form of somatic dominance'.

9 Taken from Melanie Cooper (2018) 'Yoga Adjustments.' In Sian O'Neill (ed.) Yoga Teaching Handbook: A Practical Guide for Yoga Teachers and Trainees. London and Philadelphia, PA: Singing Dragon.

10 Taken from 'Four tips for ditching yoga speak and finding your voice.' Yoga International. Available at https://yogainternational.com/article/view/4-tips-for-ditching-yoga-speak-and-finding-your-voice

11 See www.youtube.com/watch?v=J8PQjfgU8s4

Chapter 4

1 Donna Farhi (2006) Teaching Yoga: Ethics and the Teacher–Student Relationship. Berkeley, CA: Rodmell Press.

2 For more on transference, counter-transference and projection, see Donna Farhi (2006) Teaching Yoga: Ethics and the Teacher–Student Relationship. Berkeley, CA: Rodmell Press.

3 Theresa Elliott (2015) 'After 27 years teaching yoga, I got a job at the mall.' Seattle Yoga News. Available at https://seattleyoganews.com/theresa-elliott-burn-out-from-teaching-yoga-

4 Ibid.

5 See www.suzylamplugh.org/Pages/Category/national-stalking-helpline

6 You can find the Code, together with Judith Lasater's statement, in various places online, including at www.yogalifeinstitute.com/wp-content/uploads/2010/10/California-Yoga-Teachers-Association-Code-of-Conduct.pages_.pdf

7 Donna Farhi (2006) Teaching Yoga: Ethics and the Teacher–Student Relationship. Berkeley, CA: Rodmell Press.

8 Kylea Taylor (1995) The Ethics of Caring: Honouring the Web of Life in Our Professional Healing Relationships, 2nd edn. Santa Cruz, CA: Hanford Mead Publishers.

9 Theo Wildcroft (2016) 'Trauma sensitive.' Wild Yoga, 24 March. Available at www.wildyoga.co.uk/2016/03/trauma-sensitive

Chapter 5

1   It is beyond the scope of this book to discuss historical abuse in yoga. For information and a discussion of this subject, see, in particular, Matthew Remski (2019) *Practice and All Is Coming: Abuse, Cult Dynamics, and Healing in Yoga and Beyond.* Rangiora, New Zealand: Embodied Wisdom Publications.

2   www.andygill.yoga

3   For more on working with hypermobile students, see Jess Glenny (2013) 'Hypermobility on the yoga mat: Some pointers for teaching yoga to hypermobile people.' Jess's practice blog, 5 June. Available at http://movingprayer.wordpress.com/2013/06/05/teaching-yoga-to-people-with-hypermobility

4   The whole article is well worth a read: 'Safe Space.' insideowl blog, 24 August 2015. Available at www.insideowl.com/2015/08/24/safe-space

5   J. Brown (2012) 'Does studying anatomy make yoga safer?' *Yoga Therapy Today.* Available at www.jbrownyoga.com/articles/does-studying-anatomy-make-yoga-safer/

6   Personal communication.

7   'Yoga for anxiety and depression.' Harvard Mental Health Letter, April 2009. Available at www.health.harvard.edu/mind-and-mood/yoga-for-anxiety-and-depression

8   N. Gangadhar Bangalore and Shivarama Varambally (2012) 'Yoga therapy for schizophrenia.' *International Journal of Yoga* 5, 2, 85–91. Available at www.ncbi.nlm.nih.gov/pmc/articles/PMC3410202

9   There's more writing about this on my blog. See Jess's practice blog. Available at https://movingprayer.wordpress.com

10 https://youtu.be/zhHhWEFD98g

11 Chelsea Roff (2012) 'Starved for Connection: Healing Anorexia through Yoga.' In Carol Horton and Rosanne Harvey (eds) 21st Century Yoga: Culture, Politics and Practice (pp.73–94). Chicago, IL: Kleio Books. More resources are available at www.eatbreathethrive.org

12 William J. Broad (2012) 'How yoga can wreck your body.' *The New York Times*, 5 January. Available at www.nytimes.com/2012/01/08/magazine/how-yoga-can-wreck-your-body.html?_r=2&pagewanted=all

13 Quoted in J. Brown (2012) 'Does studying anatomy make yoga safer?' *Yoga Therapy Today.* Available at www.jbrownyoga.com/articles/does-studying-anatomy-make-yoga-safer/

14 Private communication.

15 Gregor Maehle (2018) 'Ashtanga's flawed teacher accreditation process.' Chintamani Yoga, 9 June. Available at http://chintamaniyoga.com/teaching/ashtangas-flawed-teacher-accreditation-process

16 http://lesliehowardyoga.com

17 Karen Miscall-Bannon (2014) 'Where do we go from here?' 24 April. Available at https://karenmiscallbannon.blogspot.com/2014/04/where-do-we-go-from-here.html

18 Quoted in Shannon Sexton (2014) 'Healing heartbreak: A yoga practice to get through grief.' *Yoga Journal*, 13 October. Available at www.yogajournal.com/lifestyle/healing-heartbreak-yoga-practice-get-grief

Chapter 6

1   https://openfloor.org/members/andrea-juhan-ph-d

2   www.donnafarhi.co.nz/wp

3   Donna Farhi (2017) 'Embracing vulnerability is the most powerful yoga.' Body Mind Love blog. YogaUOnline. Available at www.yogauonline.com/yogau-wellness-blog/donna-farhi-embracing-vulnerability-most-powerful-yoga

4   Ibid.

5   Rates of hypermobility and symptoms of autonomic dysfunction are particularly high in adults with neurodevelopmental diagnoses. It is likely that the importance of hypermobility and autonomic dysfunction to the generation and maintenance of psychopathology in neurodevelopmental disorders is poorly appreciated. See J. Eccles, V. Iodice, N. Dowell *et al.* 'Joint Hypermobility and Autonomic Hyperactivity: Relevance to Neurodevelopmental Disorders.' *Journal of Neurology, Neurosurgery and Psychiatry 85, 8.*

6 For more about teaching yoga to hypermobile people, see Jess Glenny (2013) 'Hypermobility on the yoga mat: Some pointers for teaching yoga to hypermobile people.' Jess's practice blog, 5 June. Available at http://movingprayer.wordpress.com/2013/06/05/teaching-yoga-to-people-with-hypermobility

7 www.traumasensitiveyoga.com – London TCTSY trainings are hosted by The Yoga Clinic, which has an online register of TCTSY teachers internationally: www.theyogaclinic.co.uk

8 For more about working with autistic people, see Jess Glenny (2014) 'Autistic movers and shakers: Some suggestions for supporting autistic people in yoga, dance and moving practice.' Jess's practice blog, 13 March. Available at http//movingprayer.wordpress.com/2014/03/13/autistic-movers-and-shakers-some-suggestions-for-supporting-autistic-people-in-yoga-and-moving-body-practice

9 See Jess Glenny (2014) 'Autistic movers and shakers: Some suggestions for supporting autistic people in yoga, dance and moving practice.' Jess's practice blog, 13 March. Available at http//movingprayer.wordpress.com/2014/03/13/autistic-movers-and-shakers-some-suggestions-for-supporting-autistic-people-in-yoga-and-moving-body-practice

Chapter 7

1 Quoted in Rina Raphael (2017) 'How this "fat femme" yoga instructor is reshaping the $3 trillion wellness industry.' Fast Company, 14 June. Available at www.fastcompany.com/40429705/how-this-fat-femme-yoga-instructor-is-reshaping-the-3-trillion-wellness-industry

2 In this chapter, I have chosen to use identity-first rather than person-first language ('disabled person' rather than 'person with a disability') because this is the preference of the disability rights movement. When teaching disabled students, respect their own choices in this regard. If they prefer person-first language in relation to themselves, use that.

3 Quoted in Nick Levine (2016) 'Why this LGBTQ+ yoga class is so necessary.' Evening Standard, 10 November. Available at www.standard.co.uk/lifestyle/health/why-this-queer-and-trans-yoga-class-is-so-necessary-a3392806.html

4 Jane Fae (2015) 'Which gender toilet does a trans person use? Why does it matter?' Independent, 16 January. Available at www.independent.co.uk/voices/comment/which-gender-toilet-does-a-trans-person-choose-why-does-it-matter-9983727.html

5 Rhi (2017) 'Autism awareness: Be aware of our existence.' The Mighty, 29 March. Available at https://themighty.com/2017/03/autism-awareness-be-aware-of-our-existence

6 Dianne Bondy (no date) 'Yoga, equity and social justice.' Yoga International. Available at https://yogainternational.com/article/view/yoga-equity-and-social-justice

7 Nick Krieger (2014) 'Why trans and queer yoga?' Decolonizing Yoga, 24 August, Available at www.decolonizingyoga.com/trans-queer-yoga

8 Tynan Rhea (2017) '8 gender-neutral birth terms and how to use them.' TynanRhea.com blog, 13 February. Available at www.tynanrhea.com/single-post/2017/02/13/8-gender-neutral-birth-terms-and-how-to-use-them

9 Quoted in Caroline Thompson (2017) 'Fat-positive activists explain what it's really like to be fat.' Vice, 4 May. Available at www.vice.com/en_us/article/gvzx94/fat-positive-activists-explain-what-its-really-like-to-be-fat

10 'Is is ok to call fat people fat?' Dances with Fat, 22 October 2018. Available at https://danceswithfat.wordpress.com/2018/10/22/is-it-ok-to-call-fat-people-fat

11 Quoted in Rosalie Murphy (2014) 'Why your yoga class is so white.' The Atlantic, 8 July. Available at www.theatlantic.com/national/archive/2014/07/why-your-yoga-class-is-so-white/374002

12 See Mark Singleton (2010) Yoga Body: The History of Modern Posture Practice. Oxford: Oxford University Press.

13 Kudos goes to Triyoga here, which, at the time of writing, offers disabled concessions on production of a Disabled Identification (DID) card, available to disabled people whether or not they are able to access disability benefits.

14 Quoted in Kayleen Shaefer (2015) 'They're not afraid to say it: Fat yoga.' The New York Times, 15 April 2015. Available at www.nytimes.com/2015/04/16/fashion/theyre-not-afraid-to-say-it-fat-yoga.html

15 Tiffany Kell (2013) 'Project Bendypants: Practising yoga while fat.' Decolonizing Yoga, 17 May. Available at www.decolonizingyoga.com/project-bendypants-practicing-yoga-while-fat

16 Here are a few to get you started: Anna Guest-Jelley (2013) '6 tips for teaching curvy yoga students.' Decolonizing Yoga, 5 May. Available at www.decolonizingyoga.com/6-tips-for-teaching-curvy-yoga-students; Michael Hayes (2015) '6 tips for teaching yoga to plus-size students.' Yoga Journal, 20 April. Available at www.yogajournal.com/teach/6-tips-teaching-yoga-plus-size-students; Amber Karnes (2012) 'Sun Salutation (Surya Namaskar) yoga modifications for plus-size/larger bodies.' YouTube, 22 March. Available at www.youtube.com/watch?v=IE1cz0WSZpQ

17 Anna Guest-Jelley (2017) 'How standing out in a room of skinny yogis spurred this teacher's body acceptance.' Yoga Journal, 28 April. Available at www.yogajournal.com/lifestyle/standing-out-skinny-yogis-spurred-body-acceptance

18 Quoted in Kayleen Shaefer (2015) 'They're not afraid to say it: Fat yoga.' The New York Times, 15 April 2015. Available at www.nytimes.com/2015/04/16/fashion/theyre-not-afraid-to-say-it-fat-yoga.html

19 Jagger Blaec (2016) 'What it's like being the fat girl in yoga class.' Greatist, 7 September. Available at https://greatist.com/live/what-its-like-being-the-fat-girl-at-yoga

20 See Matthew's book about his paralysis and discovery of yoga – Matthew Sanford (2008) Waking: A Memoir of Trauma and Transcendence. Emmaus, PA: Rodale Press. See also www.matthewsanford.com

21 Matthew Sanford (2008) 'I don't overcome my body; I adapt yoga to my body.' Yoga International, April. Available at https://yogainternational.com/article/view/i-dont-overcome-my-body-i-adapt-yoga-to-my-body

22 https://youtu.be/d4VjECv_YuM

23 Deaf with a capital D is used as an identifier by Deaf people who regard their deafness as a difference rather than an impairment and who identify with the language and culture of Deaf people.

24 Shakti Bell, 'Why teaching with a disability makes you an invaluable teacher.' Yoga International. Available at https://yogainternational.com/article/view/why-teaching-with-a-disability-makes-you-an-invaluable-teacher

25 See Chapter 6, note 5.

26 Jess Glenny (2013) 'Hypermobility on the yoga mat: Some pointers for teaching yoga to hypermobile people.' Jess's practice blog, 5 June. Available at http://movingprayer.wordpress.com/2013/06/05/teaching-yoga-to-people-with-hypermobility

27 Jess Glenny (2014) 'Autistic movers and shakers: Some suggestions for supporting autistic people in yoga, dance and moving practice.' Jess's practice blog, 13 March. Available at http//movingprayer.wordpress.com/2014/03/13/autistic-movers-and-shakers-some-suggestions-for-supporting-autistic-people-in-yoga-and-moving-body-practice

28 Naomi Jacobs (2017) 'Listen to our experience: On epistemic invalidation.' Lighthouse, 26 June. Available at https://butlighthouse.wordpress.com/2017/06/26/listen-to-our-experience-on-epistemic-invalidation

29 Mia Mingus is a stunning writer, and a subtle and sensitive thinker, who is well worth seeking out. Mia Mingus (2019) 'Access intimacy, interdependence and disability justice.' Leaving Evidence, 9 January. Available at https://leavingevidence.wordpress.com

30 Dianne Bondy (no date) 'Yoga, equity and social justice.' Yoga International. Available at https://yogainternational.com/article/view/yoga-equity-and-social-justice

31 www.unfoldportland.com

Chapter 8

1 https://yogatax.co.uk/help/pensions-and-retirement
2 Personal communication.
3 Richard Freeman and Mary Taylor, www.facebook.com/richardfreemanyoga
4 David Garrigues (no date) 'The bravest thing a yogi can do is to grow old and keep practising.' Available at https://davidgarrigues.com/writings/the-brave-aging-yogi
5 www.reviews.com/best-yoga-mat

6   Apparently, the major benefit of gin in the context of yin yoga is that: 'In order to target these yin tissues we must first learn to relax the surrounding muscles. A small amount of alcohol can help achieve the desired physiological state to facilitate this action.' Unfortunately, the kind of relaxation attained through alcohol is of a wholly different kind from the relaxation we're aiming for in embodied practice, which is one of heightened proprioception, interoception and connection with the body – rather than slurred speech and falling over, which is what we generally get from alcohol. As yoga teachers, we are engaged in enabling our students to regulate their own nervous system without recourse to uppers and downers. Seriously, if you need a gin to relax, you have a problem. (The class was sold out, by the way.)

7   Ruth Whippman (2018) 'Everything is for sale now. Even us.' *The New York Times*, 24 November. Available at www.nytimes.com/2018/11/24/opinion/sunday/gig-economy-self-promotion-anxiety. html?fbclid=IwAR05lQNYUENKi6S5MC8UCBICofUZEPQeB8aMbEATLP25uuoXybdisUXRKTs

8   Quoted in Brittany Risher (2017) '10 business secrets to starting a successful yoga career.' *Yoga Journal*, 11 July. Available at www.yogajournal.com/teach/10-business-secrets-to-starting-a-successful-yoga-career

9   Quoted in Risher (2017), ibid.

10   Norman Blair (2012) 'Broken gods, breaking hearts: Pedestals, boundaries, pitfalls.' Available at www.yogawithnorman.co.uk/space/1ff1de774005f8da13f42943881c655f/pdfs/brokengodsbreakinghearts_1.pdf

11   See Matthew Remski (2019) *Practice and All Is Coming: Abuse, Cult Dynamics, and Healing in Yoga and Beyond.* Rangiora, New Zealand: Embodied Wisdom Publications.

12   Personal communication.

13   Theresa Elliott (2015) 'After 27 years teaching yoga, I got a job at the mall.' *Seattle Yoga News.* Available at https://seattleyoganews.com/theresa-elliott-burn-out-from-teaching-yoga-seattle

14   You can download this at https://healing-space.teachable.com/p/healing-space-bucket

15   Jess Glenny (2013) 'Hypermobility on the yoga mat: Some pointers for teaching yoga to hypermobile people.' Jess's practice blog, 5 June. Available at http://movingprayer.wordpress.com/2013/06/05/teaching-yoga-to-people-with-hypermobility

16   Rosie Spinks (2017) 'How to politely decline giving professional advice for free.' Quartz at Work, 28 December. Available at https://qz.com/work/1166310/how-to-say-no-to-people-who-ask-for-free-advice

17   Personal communication.

Chapter 9

1   Taken from Richard Freeman and Mary Taylor, www.facebook.com/richardfreemanyoga

Index

Mysore teaching
    apprenticing and assisting 250–1
    classes of one's own, establishing 56
    room 90, 91, 133, 147, 154, 225, 236–7,
        251
    see also ashtanga vinyasa yoga

Namaskaram (IYN publication) 38
neurodiversity 208–209
    sensory environments 44
    unidentified 209–211
    see also autistic spectrum disorders
        (ASDs)
noise levels 52
nonordinary states of consciousness 131

obesity 199–200
one-to-one sessions 139, 140
online groups 110, 252
othering 196
own classes, setting up *see* classes of one's
    own, establishing
own practice, maintaining 63–4

packer (prosthetic penis) 172
pain, honouring 147–8
Palmer, Parker J. 30, 255
paralysis 207
paranoia 160–1
PAR-Q (Physical Activity Readiness
    Questionnaire) 57
Pattabhi Jois, S.K. 233, 234
pauses, honouring 82–3, 97
    in breath cycle 76, 96
payment *see* fees; financial issues
'peak' poses, letting go of 92
peer network as teacher 232–3
pelvic floor, reference to 170–1, 173
permission cards 135
permission to adjust, asking 43, 86–8,
    134–5
    see also adjustment/touch; yoga teacher–
        student relationship
phone numbers 123–4
Polivoda, C. 199
positive statements 71, 74

post-traumatic stress disorder (PTSD) 57,
    84
postures
    abandoning 148
    adjusting 35–7, 85–7, 102, 134, 166
    'advanced' 16, 109–110, 153, 179, 180
    approaching 41–2, 158
    in ashtanga vinyasa style 25, 134
    and body parts 172, 173
    breaking down 157
    contraindications 60
    dyspraxic students 209
    embodying 91, 135, 181
    external rotation 59
    fear in 145–7
    foundational architecture 72, 85
    full 147–8
    gymnastic 147, 225
    ideal website appearance 216
    key aspects 89
    language use 74, 76
        names, remembering 25
        Sanskrit, use of 25
        structure, articulating 64
    modifications *see* modifications
    'peak' poses, letting go of 92, 165
    physical alignment 148
    props 19, 211
    risk-taking 145, 172
    selecting 83
    sensation, feeling 81
    supine, passive or restorative 19, 20–1,
        93, 167, 238
        yin style 73, 76, 80, 127, 158, 260
    taking time to teach 170
    teaching without demonstrating 90–1
    templates 72
POTS (postural orthostatic tachycardia
    syndrome) 58, 91
practice communities, creating 236–7
practice of yoga
    asana practice 20–1
    defining personal meaning of yoga 243–4
    maintaining one's own practice 63–4
    practice communities, creating 236–7
    risks of 164–5
    scope of 136–9, 152–3
    transformative effect 148–50